The

COMPLETE
DIABETES
LIFESTYLE

The
COMPLETE DIABETES LIFESTYLE

Donna Kay with Maribeth Stephens

Big Think Media, Inc.

Printed in the United States of America.

For information, visit us at Big Think Media, Inc., www.bigthinkmedia.com, or contact us at info@bigthinkmedia.com

Cover and book design by Katy Scott, www.katyscott.com
Donna Kay's photograph by Susan McSpadden, www.susanmcspadden.com
Maribeth Stephens' photograph © 2007 Ingrid Pape-Sheldon, www.pape-sheldon.com

ISBN-10   0-9788108-1-3
ISBN-13   978-0-9788108-1-8

Trade names of products are properties of their respective companies, and no consideration was either given or received in exchange. Products discussed in the book should not be construed as endorsement.

Although we strive to present only current and accurate information, readers should not consider it as professional advice, which can only be given by a healthcare provider. The views and opinions expressed in these pages are those of the authors. Although great care has been taken in compiling and checking the information given in this publication to ensure accuracy, the authors, Big Think Media, Inc., and its servants or agents shall not be responsible or liable in any way for the currency of the information or for any errors, omissions, or inaccuracies in this title, whether arising from negligence or otherwise howsoever or for any consequences arising therefrom.

The information you find in this book is not intended to be medical advice and does not specifically address any particular person's health care or other needs. It should not be used in place of a visit, call, consultation with, or advice of your own physician or other health care provider. If you have any health care-related questions or concerns, please call or see your health care provider promptly. You should never disregard medical advice or delay in seeking medical advice because of something you read here.

This book is dedicated to the millions of people around the world with type 2 diabetes who make a choice every day to live a great life.

—DK

For Jim.

—MBS

ACKNOWLEDGMENTS

Donna Kay

I am so blessed to have a support system that not only helped to create this book but also helps me to have a great life. I thank my parents, whose love never waivers. I thank my husband, Geoff, and my bonus boys, Alexander and Harrison. They make life both fun and fulfilling. Thank you Lisa Mildenhall for being an all around great person. Special thanks as well to the Rasmussens (Jon, Will, and Alan), the Calcaras (Kathy, Mickey, Emily, Isabelle, Mike, and Betty) and the Copelands (Karen, Robert, Andrew, and Kate). My family members range in ages from one to eighty, and I love each and every one of you.

To Mr. William Hansey and Mr. Robert G. Crain, thank you for your solid advice, your constant support, and most of all, your belief in me.

To the three Julies: Julie Hay, Julie Sams-Naggar, and Julie Quattro. Thank you. Joan Geraghty and Lorraine Silva, you each fit the definition of a wonderful friend, and I thank you.

A virtual team of professionals helped with this project. Special thanks to Robert Killian, M.D., Bradd Silver, M.D., Betty Franke, Teresa Allen, Doug Liner, and Marc Mason.

To my coauthor, Maribeth Stephens: It is no exaggeration to say that without you, this book would not have been written. Maribeth, I thank you. We did it!

Special thanks to the publication and production team for this book, led by the amazing Arushi Sinha, Ph.D. Also thanks to Dan Fernandez, Katy Scott, Bruce Ré, and Deborah Shouse.

Last but not least, I want to thank all my friends and colleagues who took time out of their day to keep good thoughts for both me and my project. Karma is a wonderful thing, and I greatly appreciate every small positive thought on my behalf.

Maribeth Stephens

I'm convinced that books are living things. Each of the books I've had the privilege of working on, it seems, is imprinted with a unique DNA of sorts. First, the visible parts of a book are shaped by contributors who generously share both their learned knowledge and earned wisdom. Thank you, Donna, for being so open about your struggles, triumphs, questions and hopes, and letting me be the one to tell your story. I'm honored. My thanks, too, to the medical reviewers: Rob Killian, M.D., and Bradd Silver, M.D. To Ina Roy-Faderman, M.D., Ph.D., your successes are an inspiration. Thanks for sharing the wisdom that only you could provide. Thanks to certified diabetes educators Teresa Allen and Doug Liner, who make sage advice easy to understand. To Deborah Shouse, thanks for seeing what needed to go and what was worth keeping. Dan Fernandez and Suzanne Miller, thank you for providing the final polish these words needed. Bows of acknowledgement and appreciation to Christy Graunke for making things very easy to find in this book. Hats off to Katy Scott; you're a visual whiz. Arushi Sinha, Ph.D., thank you for understanding our vision and putting together such a terrific team to make it real.

A book also has invisible parts created through intangible but vital things such as connection, guidance, encouragement, and influence. Beth Likens, without you making the first connection with Donna, no one would be holding this particular work in their hands. Thank you.

Bill Broderick, Jennifer Davidson, Gail Fairfield, Valorie Fanger, Rudy Garza, Bea Kumasaka, Julie Linde, Laura Mansfield, Marie Manuchehri, Bruce Plotkin, Karen Smith, and Kathleen Toguchi: Your individual and collective guidance, encouragement, friendship, and influence run deep.

And to Jim Lindler: Words can't even begin to cover everything I have to thank you for. You're my forever.

TABLE OF CONTENTS

INTRODUCTION

How in the world did I end up with type 2 diabetes? When I was first diagnosed, that question created a continual hum in the back of my mind. Arising before me were mountains of uncertainty about what to do next. And yet everywhere I turned for help, I was left with more questions than answers.

Since those early days, though, my thinking has evolved and the hum has quieted. Now it's easy for me to own up to the fact that I *do have* diabetes, and I have to deal with it every day. It took about a year for me to get a better handle on my disease and lifestyle changes. In hindsight, I was really frustrated that my diabetes management was not easier during those first 12 months. There was no clear path for me to follow.

In my early days, I wished for a guide like this. That's my motivation for creating this book. My goal is to help you understand that with an open mind and an open heart, you have the power to change. Diabetes is not the end of the world. True, you will have to change some behaviors, but you *can* do it. Behind all the official recommendations and medical advice, there are personal stories of accomplishment and triumph. My story is one of them. And yours can be, too. When you mix the fact that you have diabetes with practical knowledge and a sense of humor, it is not all bad. In fact, I'm living better and am happier than I thought I could ever be.

This illness was my wake-up call. I got really clear, really fast not only on *what* I wanted but also *how* I wanted to live. Since being diagnosed, I have lost more than 40 pounds, coauthored a book, rode my bike in a century (100 mile) ride, married the man of my dreams, and inherited two glorious bonus boys (my stepsons). My life is busier and richer than ever. In the middle of everything is this disease that requires constant attention and management. And yet, through the management of diabetes, I am able to live my best life ever. At age 40, I truly believe my best years are ahead of me. If you can get your heart and mind wrapped around the fact that you have diabetes, your body will follow you wherever you take it.

While I have learned much about diabetes these past years, I am still a patient, doing the best that I can every day. I am not a medical doctor, so the information in this book is based on what has worked for me over the last four-plus years and accepted medical guidelines. While we have endeavored to provide you the relevant information in easy-to-understand language, we encourage you to begin—and continue—open communication with your diabetes healthcare team. Ask your doctor about newly available treatments, and keep your medical team updated on your progress and any changes in your health. Most importantly, do not ignore advice from your medical team or delay treatment because of information you find in this book.

Type 2 diabetes is a serious condition, but you can take control. When I was first diagnosed, I decided that this disease would not manage me. Instead, *I* would manage *it*. And as you begin your journey, I encourage you not only to arm yourself with reliable information but also to keep a positive attitude. Cultivating a positive outlook is one of the best things you can do to ensure a long, productive, and happy life, which is my wish for you.

Donna Kay
November 2007

CHAPTER 1

370—THE NUMBER THAT CHANGED MY LIFE

I should have known it was too good to be true. For the first time in my 35 years, I was eating whatever I wanted and losing weight. I was ravenous all day and recklessly indulged in all manner of food to ease my hunger. Despite eating farmhand-sized breakfasts, lunching on huge sandwiches, dining on steaks and potatoes loaded with butter and sour cream, and munching on carbohydrates and sugar the rest of the time, the weight was peeling off.

I was also wildly thirsty. The good news was that I was finally getting my daily-recommended dose of water—and then some. Drinking eight glasses of water had always felt like a chore, and not one I completed with ease. Of course, I was going to the bathroom like crazy during the day and getting up to urinate four or five times a night. Visiting the bathroom several times a night wasn't my only nighttime predicament. Cramps would seize my calf and send me six feet off the mattress.

Despite the enormous appetite, nagging thirst, and exhaustion from too little sleep, I reveled in the unexpected weight loss. I adored eating without worrying. Stepping onto the scale had become an experience I'd only dreamed about. No matter how many doughnuts, candy bars, filets mignon, and potato chips I ate, the dial went down. I wasn't just losing a couple of pounds here and there. The weight was dropping off as fast as I could turn around. I had lost 15 pounds in a month by eating like a horse. Had I found the Holy Grail—the ultimate Hershey's diet?

In the back of my mind, though, an alarm bell was ringing. Instinct urged me to go to the doctor. But I kept putting it off. I had back surgery for a herniated disk scheduled in a couple of weeks, and I figured I'd mention all of this to my doctor when I went in for the pre-surgery exam and blood test.

The minute I walked into my doctor's office, he said, "Looks like you've lost weight."

"Yes," I said, proudly. Then I divulged the details.

"Sounds like diabetes," he said.

I looked at him, unbelieving.

"I'll take your blood and run the tests for surgery. We'll also get your sugar count. I'll call you tomorrow."

The minute I walked out of his office, I dismissed our conversation about diabetes. After all, no one in my family had diabetes. I was too young for such an illness. Mentioning diabetes was just one of those things that doctors were supposed to say, just like they were supposed to tell you to eat less and exercise more.

· · · · · · · · · · · · · · · · · ·

I was in the kitchen the next morning when the phone rang. "Hi, Donna, it's Dr. Killian calling."

"What's the good word?"

"You have type 2 diabetes," he said.

I stood in the kitchen, one hand gripping the phone, the other clutching the counter. I heard the words, but what he said wasn't possible. Was it?

"Do you have any questions?" he asked.

My mind was buzzing. My internal monologue immediately took over. Did I have any questions? Well, for starters, why in the hell was this happening to me?! I didn't have any family history of diabetes. True, I was a solid 30 pounds heavier than I should have been. But my diet was so much better than it had been 10 years ago. Wasn't diabetes for old, sick people? I stared at the glass of cola I had just poured, my mind so frenzied I could not articulate a word.

Finally, I mustered a question. "What do I do first?"

"I've already called in a prescription. Start taking your new medicine today. Your blood sugar count is 370."

"Is that bad?"

"It's supposed to be around 100. We need to work on getting that number down right away."

By this time, a rivulet of what he was saying was seeping in. "Dr. Killian, just how freaked out should I be?"

"What do you mean?" he asked.

"On a scale of zero to 10—zero meaning I am lying in the fetal position, crying and incapable of movement and 10 meaning that in a few minutes I'll forget you said diabetes to me—how concerned do I need to be about this disease?"

He drew a breath and said, "You need to be a three or four. This is not so devastating that you need to be crippled by it, but diabetes needs to command your attention. It's manageable. But you're the one who has to manage it."

As I hung up the phone, all I could think was, "Damn. And I finally just lost 15 pounds."

....

I started out big, coming into the world at 9 pounds, 3 ounces. I never grew out of my baby fat. I was raised in St. Louis with two fabulous parents and three wonderful siblings. In my family, the food was healthy, homemade, and plentiful. At Thanksgiving and Christmas, our table groaned with the weight of stuffing, yams, pies, mashed potatoes, cranberry muffins, gravy, rolls, and turkey. And it wasn't just holidays when we ate terrific food. Mom, a teacher, was and is a great cook. At our table, the rule was that we had to take a bite of everything on our plates. We could also eat as much as we wanted of the foods we liked. I adored filling myself up, relishing second and third helpings, savoring the comfort of being full of Mom's delicious food. Our family wasn't wealthy, and Mom didn't often spend money on sweets or junk food. When we did get such treats, I really indulged. I remember competing with my sister, seeing who could eat Twinkies the fastest. On our yearly eight-hour drive to Iowa, Mom stocked up on junk food, and we ate away the miles. Despite her example of good cooking and healthy eating, I ended up taking after my father. My dad's a big guy. In those days, I took after him, eating and drinking what I wanted. I was blessed with height, but oooh boy, was I wide.

Kids at school rarely teased me about my size, and my weight never deterred me from sports or other activities. Though I was heavy, I always made the team. In high school, softball was my game. In college, I landed a spot on the university's team. As a sophomore, I switched to basketball. The idea of slimming down was constantly on my mind, but I never followed through.

When I wasn't playing sports, my college years were spent studying, eating, and drinking with friends. My friends and I gleefully indulged in the two major food groups closest to the heart of many U.S. college students: pizza and beer.

After graduation, I moved to Seattle at the height of the high-tech boom. I landed a good job and really liked the other twentysomethings I worked with. I toiled over my computer at least 10 hours a day, went out drinking and eating with my work pals at night, got home in the wee hours, and rolled out of bed a few hours later. I did this four or five nights a week. As my knowledge of Seattle's eateries and drinkeries expanded, so did I. I loved the luxury of having enough money to buy and eat whatever foods and sweets I wanted. I loved it so much that my weight hovered just above 240 pounds. By the time I reached my late 20s, my attitudes matured and I began to live a little quieter life. Plus, the long days and long nights were catching up with me. I've never been an early riser, and getting out of bed in the morning was getting tougher. Good thing I lived in Seattle and had instant access to the coffee culture. Mornings, I dragged myself to work, turned on the computer, and went straight to the coffee shop to buy a latté. When my energy plummeted midmorning, I returned to the coffee shop for a muffin or doughnut and another latté. My energy crashed at lunch time, but I boosted it with a burger and fries. Of course, I had an afternoon snack to shore me up and then a great dinner, followed by late night indulgences. Food was an important part of my social and personal life.

Still, spending the evening with friends drinking beer and noshing on pub food had lost its appeal. I cut back on drinking, as well as eating some of the carb-laden dinners. I dropped 20 pounds in a couple of months and felt a lot better.

Though I moderated my nightlife, I couldn't moderate the energy I needed to expend at work. The days were packed with all sorts of activity. Except exercise. Although I had been an athlete in college, after I left school, all of my athletic knowledge failed to make it from my head to my muscles. I'd get in a great exercise groove for about three weeks and then stop for months at a time. I had more unused gym memberships than I could count. I would read some new exercise program, get inspired to go the gym, and vow that this time I'd stick with a schedule. But a few weeks later I would stop.

Besides working long hours, I also traveled extensively. Being in different time zones, feeling fatigued from disturbed sleep, and attending meetings and conferences did not help me lead a balanced physical life. For many years, this lifestyle added up to eating and drinking at odd hours and rarely exercising.

When I was 30, I was laid off. For the first time in more than eight years, I had huge chunks of time for myself. Instead of going to the office every day, I went to the gym. I put into practice all the information I knew about exercise, and I modified my eating to take in five or six smaller meals a day. I felt fabulous and lost 20 pounds. But the new me ended as soon as I got a new job. My lost weight got found and I returned to my old habits—until that phone call from Dr. Killian.

REALITY BITES

I still couldn't believe it. I had diabetes. This couldn't be happening to me. It just didn't make sense. I sat at my kitchen table, numb with disbelief and fear. Finally, I pushed myself into action. I called my older sister, a nurse, and told her the news. She was as shocked as I was, and we spent 20 minutes repeating the phrase, "I can't believe it."

I called my mom and she, too, was dumbfounded. There was no family history of the illness. I asked Mom to tell my other family members. As the initial shock subsided, my desire for information grew. I began researching. I went to the bookstore and bought books on diabetes. I combed the Internet. I began learning all I could about type 2 diabetes.

Ten days after my doctor told me I had diabetes, I had a successful outpatient surgery to repair the herniated disk. I was home for about a week when a staph infection attacked the site of the incision, and I landed back in the hospital, enduring two surgeries in five days to clean everything up. While in the hospital, Dr. Killian called regularly to check on me and my diabetes. Since it was going to be a while until I was up and around, Dr. Killian decided it was then that I should start my formal diabetes education. From my early research and reading, I felt I knew some of the changes I needed to make. I'm glad he suggested that I start my diabetes education program while in the hospital because I was ready for a real discussion with someone who knew their stuff and could explain it to me. A couple of days after Dr. Killian mentioned starting inpatient diabetes education, the certified diabetes educator walked into my hospital room, pulled up a chair, and began to lecture: "Well, with diabetes, you want to watch what you eat."

She hadn't asked anything about me or my lifestyle before she launched into her routine. "After you get out of the hospital, you're going to want to exercise," she droned. I was a little taken aback. She didn't ask me any questions. She simply lectured. And this educator sounded a little like a metronome with a nasal condition. After an hour of hearing about all of the sacrifices I would have to make, I felt sentenced to a purgatory of boring regimentation. If life was going to be like this, I might as well die 30 pounds overweight and with a big chocolate smile on my lips. Maybe I was just having a bad day. After all, I was only a couple of days from getting out of the hospital and was itching to go home. Maybe the dietitian, set to come in the following day, would be more interesting. I'd always enjoyed nutritional theories as a subject. I'd never put them into practice, but I knew a lot about them. The next day, the dietitian dropped by. Like the diabetes educator, she too, pulled up a chair and launched into her speech.

"You can eat any kind of vegetable you want," she said.

The dietitian was the last person who stood between me and my discharge from the hospital, and I was feeling feisty. I couldn't let her statement go unchallenged. "What about potatoes?" I asked. "I don't think I'm supposed to have carte blanche on them because they're a starch. Right?"

"Well, yes, potatoes are considered a starch," she agreed.

I asked, "How do you count carrots? They're a vegetable, but they are high in sugar—so they'll spike your blood sugar. You're telling me to have all the vegetables I want. How do you count a serving of carrots?"

She paused, and then slowly said, "Well, a carrot would be counted as a carrot."

I was flabbergasted. The reading I had done about the glycemic index (I'll touch on that in Chapter 6) showed that a serving of cooked carrots had a high probability of rapidly increasing my blood sugar. Sure, I was new to diabetes, but I was pretty sure I wasn't supposed to be eating my fill of anything that could trigger rapid blood sugar spikes. Vegetables seemed a difficult topic, so I switched subjects. Bread is most often made of highly processed grains, which can also send the blood sugar soaring. I knew that some bread was allowed in the diabetic diet but wasn't sure how to factor it in. I was truly looking for guidance when I asked, "How should I handle bread in my diet?"

With great deliberation she stated, "A piece of bread is pretty much a piece of bread." Well, what did that mean? Was I supposed to skip bread? Could I have some with other foods? If so, how much? And when?

And that was the beginning of my diabetes education. I left the hospital brimming with questions and feeling frustrated and overwhelmed. Feeling

9

overwhelmed is one of the most common reactions for a newly diagnosed type 2 diabetes patient. Most of us can't even think about how to get through the first year with this thing; we first have to figure out how to manage the next meal. Then we have to get through the next day, followed by the next week and the next month.

Despite my early brush with disheartening diabetes education, I've learned several secrets that I want to pass on. The biggest secret is to stop thinking about getting through the first year of diabetes. Diabetes is a daily disease. I have to take steps every day. So will you. Those daily steps will also let you know that you can take control of your disease, still have fun, and remain vital and vibrant during the most productive decades of your life. Let's begin.

CHAPTER 2

JUST THE FACTS, JACK!

None of my friends had diabetes. None of my family had diabetes. I knew only one person, a co-worker, who had the condition. When I was first diagnosed, I felt so alone, so singled out. Then I began doing research and learned that more than 20 million others in the United States have some form of diabetes. The Centers for Disease Control and Prevention (CDC) reported more than 1 million U.S. adults between 18 and 79 years of age were diagnosed with diabetes in a single year. Nearly 27 percent of diabetes patients reported being under 40 years old when they were diagnosed.[1]

The United States isn't the only country struggling with the rapid increase in diabetes. According to the World Health Organization, 171 million people around the world have diabetes, and 90 percent of them have type 2. The illness is growing at an alarming rate. By the year 2025, researchers estimate that 333 million people worldwide will have diabetes.[2] So all of us with type 2 diabetes are in good company.

If your experience is anything like mine, you're wondering what this disease is and how you ended up with it. You want simple, straightforward answers in easy-to-understand language that won't take weeks of reading and rereading to understand.

BLOOD GLUCOSE: THE QUICKIE EXPLANATION

Cells in your body need fuel to function. That fuel is glucose. Glucose—a type of sugar—is formed when the carbohydrates you eat are broken down during digestion. The main role of carbohydrates is to provide energy. Your intestine breaks down carbohydrates into glucose, which is then taken up by cells to be used for energy.

Glucose doesn't get into your cells by itself. Something has to help it. Before you put gas in a car, you have to open the gas cover. Once that's open, you can pump in all the gas the tank can hold. Just like you open the cover to get the gas into your car, the something that opens the cover in your cells, so to speak, is insulin.

Insulin, a hormone, is made by the pancreas. Hormones are chemical messengers made by glands to help control activities throughout your body. Insulin is the hormone that lets cells take in glucose from your bloodstream to be used as fuel. Insulin is created by specialized cells in the pancreas, called the beta cells. (Beta cells are also written using the Greek letter for beta: β. You might see *β cells* in other materials you read, so I'm including the term here so you're familiar with it.) After you eat, beta cells can sense the rise in blood sugar levels. They then release insulin into the bloodstream. When everything is working just right, insulin ushers the glucose inside the body's cells. But in type 2 diabetes, something is amiss. Perhaps the beta cells don't make enough insulin to handle all of the glucose in the bloodstream. Or the cells don't respond to insulin so the glucose can't get into the cells; this is called insulin resistance. For a while, the pancreas can work to produce more insulin to get the glucose into the cells that need it. Over time, though, the pancreas can slowly shut down insulin production altogether.

With so much glucose circulating, two problems occur. First, cells in the body are starved for energy, which is why diabetes is sometimes referred to as starvation in the midst of plenty. Secondly, over time, the high level of glucose can cause serious damage to the nerves, eyes, kidney, heart, and blood vessels (Chapter 9).

OTHER TYPES OF DIABETES

There are several different kinds of diabetes. Besides type 2 diabetes, there are two other commonly diagnosed forms of diabetes: type 1 and gestational.

TYPE 1 DIABETES

This is also known as insulin-dependent diabetes mellitus. It used to be called *juvenile diabetes*. It's usually first diagnosed in children, teenagers, or young adults. Type 1 diabetes develops because the body fails to produce insulin. In type 1 diabetes, the beta cells that create the insulin cannot produce it because the immune system—the body's complex network that fights infection, battles disease, and protects against invading viruses and bad bacteria—has mistaken beta cells as something harmful and has attacked and destroyed them. Researchers aren't sure why this happens, but they think that heredity (the transmission of characteristics from one generation to the next) has something to do with it. In the majority of cases, people with type 1 diabetes inherited the risk factors from both parents.

GESTATIONAL DIABETES

Gestational diabetes only occurs in pregnant women. It's found in moms-to-be who have never had diabetes but whose blood sugar levels are high during pregnancy. It affects fewer than 5 percent of pregnant women. The cause of gestational diabetes is unclear, but researchers have some leads. The placenta, which supports the baby as it develops inside the mother's body, creates a large number of hormones needed for the baby's growth. But these hormones can also interfere with the mother's ability to use insulin, thus leading to diabetes. Gestational diabetes usually goes away after the birth of the baby. But once a mother has it, the chances are high—about two out of three—that diabetes will reappear in future pregnancies. Doctors have also found that type 2 diabetes often develops years later in many women who had gestational diabetes.

WHAT CAUSES TYPE 2 DIABETES?

Researchers are a little at odds about exactly how and why type 2 diabetes develops, but they have reached some common ground about what contributes to it. The general factors are genetics, lifestyle, and age.

The genetics factor

As with type 1 diabetes, genes play an important role in whether or not a person develops type 2 diabetes. In fact, family history of type 2 diabetes is one of the strongest indicators of the potential for developing the condition. Though obese people are three to five times more likely to develop diabetes compared to those of normal weight, type 2 diabetes is also diagnosed in people whose weight is normal. And many who are obese don't develop diabetes.[3] This is why researchers think genes play a big part.

Some researchers think that the genes that may play some part in influencing the development of diabetes are the so-called *thrifty genes*. It's thought that these inherited genes let your body use food very efficiently. This means you can gain weight eating less food while others without the thrifty genes can eat plates full of carbs without tipping the scales.

The thrifty genes, great at converting energy to fat and storing it up for later use, probably helped your ancestors survive eons ago when food was much scarcer than it is today. But thrifty genes and our Western lifestyle, with its fat-laden food and sedentary way of life, don't mix particularly well. Because they're great at helping to store fat, thrifty genes likely mean that people can eat normal amounts of food but add weight. In turn, being overweight creates a higher risk for developing type 2 diabetes.

Lifestyle dangers

Type 2 diabetes develops mostly in those living a Western lifestyle—which these days means eating too much fat, too few complex carbohydrates, too little fiber, and getting too little exercise. As our collective weight has gone up, so has the number of diagnosed cases of type 2 diabetes. Excess weight encourages insulin resistance. Remember, insulin resistance means that your cells have trouble using insulin, and insulin is the key that lets blood sugar into the cells to be used as fuel.

It's not only excess weight but also where the weight settles. People who have central body obesity—carrying extra weight above the hips—are at greater risk of developing type 2 diabetes than those whose extra weight rests on the hips and thighs.

While excess weight increases the chance of developing type 2 diabetes, not everyone who is overweight will develop the illness. In fact, sometimes excess weight doesn't play a role at all. Even the slender among us can end up with type 2 diabetes.

The age aspect

Advancing age is a risk factor for developing type 2 diabetes, too. About half of the new cases of type 2 diabetes tend to occur in people 55 and older. While it's not crystal clear why more cases of diabetes are diagnosed as people age, researchers note that many older people are overweight, and excess weight is a risk factor for type 2 diabetes.

Prediabetes

Before you developed type 2 diabetes, you likely had *prediabetes*. That is, your blood sugar levels were higher than normal but not high enough to be identified as diabetes.

There are two types of prediabetes. The first is impaired fasting glucose, or IFG. Basically, IFG means that your blood sugar is too high after you have not eaten for at least eight hours. When you wake up in the morning, or otherwise haven't eaten for several hours, blood sugar is usually below 100 mg/dL. (The measurement used to indicate the amount of glucose in a set amount of blood is known as *milligrams per deciliter*, abbreviated as mg/dL.) In IFG, the blood sugar is higher than normal (100–125 mg/dL) after an overnight fast, but not high enough to be considered diabetes.

Impaired glucose tolerance (IGT) is the second type of prediabetes. Here, the blood sugar is higher (140–199 mg/dL) after an oral glucose test, in which blood glucose levels are tested after drinking a specific kind of sugary drink.

THE NUMBERS IN A NUTSHELL[4]

FASTING PLASMA GLUCOSE TEST	DIAGNOSIS
Below 100 mg/dL	Normal
100–125 mg/dL	Prediabetes (impaired fasting glucose)
Above 125 mg/dL	Diabetes
ORAL GLUCOSE TOLERANCE TEST	DIAGNOSIS
Below 140 mg/dL	Normal
140–199 mg/dL	Prediabetes (impaired glucose tolerance)
Above 199 mg/dL	Diabetes

If you're reading this book, chances are you or someone you know has already been diagnosed with type 2 diabetes. Or you may have friends or loved ones who have been warned by a doctor that they have prediabetes. You can be of immense help by telling them to take action to manage their blood glucose now so they can delay or prevent type 2 diabetes from developing. The Diabetes Prevention Program (DPP) study[5] found that people with prediabetes can prevent the development of type 2 diabetes by changing what they eat and increasing their physical activity. This study was designed to look at whether diet and exercise or a particular drug could prevent or delay the onset of type 2 diabetes. More than 3,200 people with prediabetes were randomly assigned to different groups. The first group received extensive information about diet, exercise, and behavior modification. Their goal was to reduce their weight by 7 percent and exercise at least 150 minutes per week. Members of the second group took a medication to help reduce their blood sugar levels. They also received information on diet and exercise, but they did not receive intensive counseling efforts like the first group.

The first group (the diet-and-exercise group) reduced the chance of developing diabetes by a whopping 58 percent. The second group (the medication group) also reduced the chance of developing diabetes, but by only 31 percent. This study clearly showed that eating better and getting more exercise played an even bigger role in decreasing the chances of developing type 2 diabetes than just taking a drug.

Turning Knowledge to Action

I'm glad I took the time to understand the mechanics of blood sugar and insulin because it made me feel like I had more control in the matter and less like a victim. And knowledge—along with a good bit of trial and error as I was starting out—has been the key in learning to manage this illness and live my best possible life. Now that you know the basics, you can begin to manage your own diabetes and develop a new positive attitude, which is what I call a type 2 attitude.

CHAPTER 3

TAKING MEASURE

A fter my diagnosis, I realized that I was lucky. I had a team of people with me when I performed my first blood sugar test at home. My mom and two sisters were visiting, helping me recover from back surgery. We all went to the store to select a blood glucose monitor. I didn't know what I was doing or what I should be looking for. But a particularly memorable television commercial stuck with me, so I picked up that brand of meter when we went shopping.

Once home, we settled around the dining room table. My older sister, the nurse, took the kit apart, read the directions, figured out how it worked, and then tested her own blood sugar.

"I want to know what you're going to be doing every day," she told me. "I want to experience this."

Her words gave me a sense of calm and comfort. I felt so loved when my younger sister also tested her blood sugar. Then it was my turn. As I pricked myself, I thought, "I can't believe I have to stick myself several times every day for the rest of my life." My mom, a little reluctantly, also tested her blood sugar. With my family so supportive, I felt really encouraged to make this part of my everyday life.

For the first couple of weeks, it was fascinating to test my blood sugar and see the numbers ebb and flow throughout the day. After two weeks, the thrill was gone. To keep it interesting, I turned it into a game, guessing what my blood sugar would be. My doctor had told me to test a couple of times a day. But later, when I found an endocrinologist and a team dedicated to diabetes management, I learned that if I wanted to manage my diabetes well, I would probably have to test six to ten times a day. I tested this often because I needed to know where my blood sugar was and if I needed to make changes. If my number was too high, I could get out and walk for a half hour. If it was too low, I could eat a little something.

THE POWER OF DAILY TESTING

One of the most important acts you're going to perform today, tomorrow, and all of the tomorrows after that, is to measure your blood sugar. Daily blood sugar measurements give you a snapshot of what's happening with your diabetes right now, as well as the information you need to live a balanced and healthy life. I have found that testing six to ten times a day is right for me. It could be right for you, too. But be sure to talk with your own doctor or diabetes educator about how frequently you should test. The ultimate goal of any person with diabetes is to achieve strong blood sugar control. You can't control it if you don't measure and understand your spikes, drops, and longer-term trends.

BLOOD SUGAR TARGETS

Monitoring your blood sugar is one of the best tools to track your diabetes, for both you and your healthcare team. When you share a log of blood sugar readings with your physician, you both will have a clear picture of how your body is reacting to your diabetes management plan.

RECOMMENDED BLOOD SUGAR RANGES

AMERICAN DIABETES ASSOCIATION[6]	
Plasma glucose before meals (preprandial)	90–130 mg/dL
Plasma glucose after meals (postprandial)	less than 180 mg/dL
AMERICAN COLLEGE OF ENDOCRINOLOGY[7]	
Fasting plasma glucose	less than 110 mg/dL
Postprandial blood glucose	less than 140 mg/dL

This chart notes the recommended glucose levels by two of the leading diabetes authorities, the American Diabetes Association (ADA) and the American College of Endocrinology (ACE). Let's go through some of the words in the chart, starting with *plasma*. Blood is made up of many parts—liquid, cells, and cell-like particles. When you use blood pricked from your finger to test your blood sugar level, you're using all parts of your blood—whole blood—to get that reading. A laboratory, using a blood sample provided by your doctor, will base your reading on plasma in your blood. Plasma is the liquid portion of blood. It's the color of straw and contains salts and proteins along with other substances, the most important of which for our purposes is blood sugar. Plasma glucose values are about 10 to 15 percent higher than the reading you would get with whole blood.

You'll also notice *prandial* in the chart. It's a word that simply means *related to a meal*. Pre-, of course, means before, and post- means after. So, preprandial means before a meal and postprandial means after a meal.

One of the most common questions about home kits to test blood sugar is, "Are they accurate?" In my experience, yes—as long as you use the device correctly. Usually readings are within a range of 10–15 percent of doctors' tests. Again, this is because you're using whole blood while your doctor's office is testing plasma. Regardless of whether you're looking at whole blood or plasma results, work carefully with your healthcare team to determine the blood sugar targets best for you.

TESTING TIPS

Some insurance providers will provide a blood glucose testing kit as part of your insurance benefits, so be sure to check your coverage. Many insurance companies provide partial coverage on the kits. You'll also want to look into coverage on the testing strips. My doctor wrote a prescription for the strips so I could get the insurance-discounted rate. This is important because test strips are expensive, and you will probably be using several test strips per day.

You can buy a testing kit at any drugstore and many large, one-stop retail centers. Currently, the kits are usually less than $100. These kits have well-written instructions on how to get accurate measurements. However, here are a few of the most important things I've learned about taking blood sugar measurements:

★ Wash your hands in warm water before testing. This promotes blood flow to the fingers. Also, you want clean hands when working with your lancet.

★ The lancet is a needle device that you will use to poke your finger to get the blood sample. Don't worry, it doesn't hurt very much. The slight sting afterward may last for several seconds, and up to a couple of minutes.

★ Always dispose of lancets in a home-sized hazardous container (sharps container). They are available at drugstores for just a few dollars. Once full, take the container back to the drugstore or your health clinic for disposal, because needles and lancets have special disposal requirements. The disposal fee is usually small.

★ The blood glucose reading should appear in 5–30 seconds, depending on the type of device you have. The meter you use at home will test whole blood, but some meters now can present results as *the plasma equivalent.*

★ Don't forget to record your reading in the logbook provided with the glucose monitoring kit or on another chart where you consistently keep your readings. I devised my own chart, which I'll talk more about in Chapter 7.

THE POWER OF HEMOGLOBIN A1c (HbA1c OR A1c) TESTING

If a single blood sugar reading is like a snapshot in time, then the HbA1c test is like the entire photo album of how you've been managing your blood sugar over the preceding two or three months.

Hb stands for hemoglobin, which is a protein in red blood cells. The iron in hemoglobin gives blood its red color. Hemoglobin's job is to carry oxygen from your lungs to the rest of your body's tissue. It then picks up carbon dioxide from those tissues and transports it to the lungs to be exhaled.

As glucose travels throughout the bloodstream, it's normal for blood sugar molecules to bind with a small percentage of hemoglobin. This process is called glycation. In people without diabetes, 4–6 percent of hemoglobin binds to blood sugar molecules.[7] But for people with diabetes, this percentage is naturally going to be higher because there's more glucose in the blood.

Here's a quick explanation of how the HbA1c test (often shortened to A1c) sheds a bright light on how you've been managing blood sugar over time. Hemoglobin survives for about three months, giving it an extended opportunity to hook up with glucose in the bloodstream. Since hemoglobin stays around for a good long while, looking at the percentage connected to blood sugar molecules is a terrific indicator of how well you've been managing your blood sugar over the last several weeks. Experts recommend that people with diabetes keep their HbA1c level to about 6.5 percent or less.[7] And the closer to a normal range, the better.

Let's create a hypothetical situation: About 10 weeks ago, you really had a tough time keeping your blood sugar under control. You traveled a lot for work, ate high-carb foods at odd hours, and couldn't find the time to exercise. In just the last couple of weeks, though, you've been back at home and able to stick to your eating and exercise plan. You feel better, look better, and are happy with your most recent blood glucose numbers.

You show up for your regular three-month doctor's appointment, and your physician takes a blood sample for the HbA1c test. Later, when the HbA1c results come back, it shows a higher-than-desired percentage of blood sugar molecules attached to hemoglobin. The HbA1c reading lets your doctor know that things got a little out of whack over much of the last three months. Given this information, your doctor might find out if you need some extra help, such as medication, to help keep glucose levels steady and in a healthy range.

The HbA1c test is typically done in your doctor's office but home HbA1c testing kits are on the market. These are one-time use kits, and you get results in about eight minutes. The home testing kits are convenient and relatively accurate, but they are not a substitute for regular visits to your doctor.

DIABETES MEDICATIONS

Now that you've been diagnosed with type 2 diabetes, your healthcare team will help you get started on reducing your blood sugar levels. The goal is to get them into a normal, healthy range. This is most commonly achieved through an eating and exercise plan. If lifestyle changes alone don't work, your team will probably start you on medications. There are a handful of general classes of drugs that do different things—everything from helping your muscles become more sensitive to using insulin to slowing carbohydrate absorption. Your physician will take into account factors such as your lifestyle, overall health, and personal needs in guiding you to the right prescription regimen. The chart on the next page gives a brief overview of the types of drugs and how they specifically help bring down your blood sugar. Any drug can pose a risk of serious side effects. Be sure to work closely with your healthcare team to establish and follow your unique medication plan.

EXAMPLES OF DRUGS TO HELP MANAGE TYPE 2 DIABETES

TYPE OF DRUG	ACTION	SOME BRAND NAMES	USUAL DOSES PER DAY
Alpha-Glucosidase Inhibitors	Slows digestion of carbohydrates, delays glucose absorption, reduces the level of after-meal blood glucose levels	Precose Glyset	3
Biguanides	Reduces the amount of glucose made by the liver, improves muscles' uptake and use of glucose	Glucophage	2–3
Incretin Mimetics	Stimulates insulin secretion, suppresses liver's glucose production, may help reduce appetite, slows the rate at which food exits the stomach	Byetta	2 injections
Insulin	Helps the body use blood glucose	Brand name depends on type of insulin used: rapid-, short-, intermediate-, or long-acting; premixed	The dose size and frequency must be determined by your healthcare team
Meglitinides	Stimulates insulin secretion, enhances glucose uptake in the muscles	Starlix Prandin	2–4
Sulfonylureas	Stimulates insulin secretion, decreases the liver's glucose production	Amaryl Glucotrol XL DiaBeta	1–2
Thiazolidinediones	Improves sensitivity to insulin, suppresses liver's glucose production	Avandia Actos	1–2

A NOTE ABOUT INSULIN

If diet, exercise, and oral medications have not satisfactorily reduced your blood sugar levels, your doctor may start you on insulin. For most of us with type 2 diabetes, the topic of insulin brings up fear and uncertainty. Diabetes is a progressive illness, which means that most of us, at some point, will use insulin as part of our treatment regimen. Some see starting insulin therapy as a failure to properly manage their diabetes. This is absolutely *not* the case. Insulin is a treatment and should be viewed as such. There is no shame or failure in utilizing the most appropriate treatments available to manage your diabetes.

I was able to effectively manage my blood sugar levels for quite some time with oral medication, exercise, and diet. However, after a period of time, it got harder and harder for me to keep my blood sugar numbers within a good range. Together, my doctor and I decided to add insulin to my regimen. Here are a few of the important things I've learned:

★ Insulin helps your cells to more efficiently process the nutrients you consume by way of the food you eat. In a sense, insulin helps to make every calorie count.

★ One of the biggest side effects of insulin is weight gain. People new to insulin typically enjoy the results of lower blood sugar. However, don't take this new level of control as a license to eat more (especially junk food). With insulin helping your cells to utilize every calorie, it's easy for the pounds to pile on quickly.

★ To avoid weight gain with insulin, make sure to eat a diet that is within nutritional guidelines. And don't forget to exercise 30–60 minutes a day, most days of the week.

★ Currently, most insulin treatments are still delivered by injection. The needles are thinner than a strand of human hair, and it really does not hurt. In early 2006, the U.S. Food and Drug Administration (FDA) approved for adults a powdered form of insulin that's inhaled into the lungs. But the FDA noted that it is not to be used by those who smoke or have quit smoking within the last six months. Nor is it recommended for those with other health conditions such as asthma, bronchitis, or emphysema.[8]

★ Insulin can dramatically affect your blood sugar levels. Make sure to keep your glucose meter handy and measure often. You should especially be aware of the fact that too much insulin can cause hypoglycemia, which is blood sugar that dips below 70 mg/dL. Get all of the facts from your healthcare team, and know that insulin therapy is easier than ever.

PREGNANCY AND DIABETES: A SUCCESSFUL COMBINATION

Ina Roy-Faderman, M.D., Ph.D., is a role model. She inspires others not only in her accomplished professional life as a physician, professor, and published writer, but as a woman with diabetes who has brought a healthy son into the world. Dr. Roy-Faderman has type 1 diabetes (different from gestational diabetes) and is a medical ethicist who consults for leading organizations such as the National Institute of Mental Health. Here she offers her own wisdom about managing diabetes and pregnancy.

. . . .

It can be frightening to look through information on pregnancy and diabetes; scary words and phrases like *fetal macrosomia* (a baby that's too big), birth defects and miscarriage get thrown around. So I was both surprised and relieved when my obstetrician said to me, "Your diabetes is well controlled, so we can pretty much treat this pregnancy like any other pregnancy."

By working with your diabetes, you have already unlocked the door to a healthy pregnancy for both you and your baby. By actively engaging in caring for yourself and managing your diabetes, you've got the framework for managing diabetes during pregnancy and for good prenatal care.

PLANNING FOR PREGNANCY

Just like the rest of managing your diabetes, planning is key to having a great pregnancy. Ideally, you should be working with your diabetes for three to six months before you start trying to conceive; working with your diabetes includes keeping your blood sugars within your target range.

The magic number is 7: The number and severity of birth defects in babies born to moms with diabetes drops significantly if your HbA1c is below 7 percent.

Changing medications and starting insulin: If you're currently managing your diabetes with diet and exercise, your doctor may ask you to start taking insulin to help manage your blood sugars. Pregnancy makes our bodies more resistant to insulin than usual, and taking insulin by injection helps overcome the extra resistance. If you're currently on oral medication, your doctor will want to change you over to insulin either before or as soon as you become pregnant, since most oral medications are not safe to take during pregnancy: The switch to needles can be frustrating at first, but you'll soon be taking insulin with ease.

Of course, sometimes pregnancy just happens! In that case, make sure that you seek prenatal care right away, both from an obstetrician and from your endocrinologist. Together you can create a plan to make sure that your blood sugars, HbA1c, and management program are working for the growing fetus.

DURING PREGNANCY

Managing diabetes during pregnancy will surprise you because it's so much like managing your diabetes when you're not pregnant.

Exercise is always important, but it's crucial during pregnancy. Because your body is less sensitive to insulin, you need to help your muscles use glucose to keep your blood sugars in the normal range. A 15 or 20 minute walk after each meal and snack (unless you've specifically been told by a doctor not to take walks) will help the calories you eat get to all the places they need to go to help your body do all the new activities it's engaged in. As you and your baby progress through the pregnancy, you may find that your insulin needs increase. Exercise will help you to moderate the amount of insulin you need, as well.

Morning sickness can be managed a lot like stomach flu. If you're not able to eat much in your first trimester or you vomit after eating, your insulin may need to be adjusted to keep you from having low blood sugar, which can be dangerous for you. You may also want to monitor your blood sugars and ketones more often than you might otherwise to make sure that nausea isn't impairing your health. Ketones are acids occurring from the breakdown of fat and muscle. Too many ketones can lead to a serious condition called ketoacidosis and may result in a coma. Ketoacidosis is of more concern among people with type 1 diabetes and is less common in those with type 2 diabetes. However, moms-to-be who have any type of diabetes should test for ketones.

Limited weight gain during pregnancy means a better outcome for you and your baby. Depending on your pre-pregnancy weight, you will probably need to gain less weight during the course of your pregnancy than moms without diabetes. One way to do this is to do what you've been doing with all your diabetes management: Make every calorie count. Lots of small healthy meals with few empty calories (such as refined sugar) will help keep your weight gain on track and ensure that your baby gets the nutrients he or she needs. One thing to keep in mind though: While weight loss may be part of your non-pregnancy diabetes management plan, don't try to diet during pregnancy. Moms with diabetes make ketones if not getting enough nourishment, and that can be harmful for both mom and baby. Your doctors will probably ask you to monitor the ketones in your urine by using a small strip of paper that changes color if your body is making ketones. If you're making more than trace amounts, you will want to work with your doctors and/or a nutrition specialist to help get the right diet in place.

Create a routine for taking your blood sugar frequently. You may have a chart, or you might want to tie your blood sugar checks to daily events (before and after meals, before you roll out of bed, before you brush your teeth). Since you'll be monitoring often during pregnancy, the more that it's part of your daily life, the easier it will be. Some people find that a partner or friend acting as a reminder for a frequently missed check (after lunch, for example) can also help, especially when you're busy with preparations for the new baby.

Overall, the main thing to remember is don't panic. Managing your diabetes is just another way of taking care of yourself and your baby-to-be.

—*Ina Roy-Faderman, M.D., Ph.D.*

THE DAWN EFFECT

In the beginning, my waking blood sugar levels seemed illogical. I tested my blood sugar before I went to bed, and it was 120mg/dL. When I woke up and tested before eating, it was 140 mg/dL. It didn't make sense that my sugar levels were higher after a full night of not eating rather than shortly after dinner. I asked my doctor at the time about the spike, and he didn't seem to know.

For six months, these numbers drove me crazy, until I learned about the Dawn Effect (also called the Dawn Phenomenon). In some people with diabetes, the fasting blood sugar reading (first reading of the day, before you have anything to eat or drink) is higher than the reading from the previous night. It can be worrisome, because ideally your fasting blood sugar reading should be relatively low, around 100 mg/dL. Logic alone would demand that your reading after eight hours of sleep (and therefore no food) would be lower than what it was before you went to bed.

While you are sleeping, your body releases many hormones, including those that affect blood sugar levels: glucagon, epinephrine (adrenaline), growth hormone, and cortisol. The release of these hormones is a normal function, but they can increase insulin resistance. Just before we wake, for most of us, glucose levels increase just enough to get us going. Insulin, of course, normally ushers that glucose into cells. But since these other hormones released at night can increase insulin resistance, the cells can't use that morning burst of glucose. It remains in the bloodstream. That's why the reading can be higher in the morning than when you went to bed.

There could be another reason why your blood sugar level is higher in the morning. It's called the Somogyi effect. This may occur because the blood sugar level gets too low at night. In reaction to a low blood sugar episode, the body releases glucose that's stored in the liver and muscles into the bloodstream. So the sugar is forced to remain in the bloodstream, giving you a higher blood sugar reading in the morning. A consistently higher level of morning blood sugar is a complicated issue. Be sure to tell your doctor. He or she will be able to help you understand what's causing it, as well as give excellent advice about how to manage it.

KNOW YOUR HIGHS AND LOWS

Hyperglycemia (high blood sugar) and hypoglycemia (low blood sugar) are two conditions that you will likely experience. Both have symptoms, and both can be very dangerous.

Hyperglycemia is something every person with diabetes is familiar with. When your blood sugar is too high, symptoms may include increased thirst, frequent urination, and blurry vision. If your blood sugar goes too high without treatment, you can go into a coma. Preventing such an episode is one more reason for a good diabetes management plan that includes the right foods and the right amount of exercise.

Hypoglycemia, which is defined as blood sugar at 70 mg/dL or lower, has its own set of symptoms, including shaking, dizziness, sudden weakness, hunger, and fatigue. Additionally, you may break into a sweat, have a fast heartbeat, headache, and/or a sudden mood change. If you experience these symptoms, you should eat a fast-acting carbohydrate right away: Half a cup of fruit juice, or half a can of regular soda will quickly raise your blood sugar levels, and you will usually feel more like yourself within 15 minutes. A word of caution is in order here: Some dietitians suggest that eating hard candy is not as effective as other faster-acting methods of raising blood sugar, such as a tablespoon of honey or half a can of regular soda. Hard candies may take too long to work. The general rule is, when you have hypoglycemia, eat 15 grams of fast-acting carbs, then wait 15 minutes. Check your blood sugar again, and if it has not increased to a normal level, eat another 15 grams of fast-acting carbs. Wait 15 minutes and check your blood sugar again.

Hypoglycemia can come on fast and strong. Therefore, it is important to let friends and family know the symptoms, as sometimes they may catch it before you do. With me, I am usually shaking before I realize how low my blood sugar has dropped. I always check my blood sugar before I drive, exercise, or take part in any other activity where a sudden drop in blood sugar could be particularly dangerous.

THE ULTIMATE MANAGEMENT PROJECT

Managing a staff is one of the things I love most about working in the corporate world. Yet with this illness, I've learned a whole new meaning of management. I now manage my health to the best of my ability because the best years are ahead, and I want to be able to enjoy them. As the manager of my own health, I quickly learned the importance of creating a workable routine. I understood that the better and more tightly I controlled my blood sugar levels, the better the chances of avoiding complications such as blindness and kidney failure. Though testing and management takes time, it also gives me a sense of comfort, empowerment, and wonderful health.

CHAPTER 4

YOU GOTTA HAVE FRIENDS

Normally, I like to solve my own problems. I pride myself on my independent and creative thinking, and on my ability to research and uncover solutions. But dealing with diabetes has taught me to value more deeply the knowledge and insights of others, to reach out for help when I need it, and to appreciate the wealth of having a community of caring people to call upon.

Diabetes is not a friendly disease. Unmanaged, it can take its toll physically, emotionally, financially, and perhaps even socially. That's why you need friends to help get you through.

Think back to the times when you've hit rough patches. Now think about who helped you through—it was probably more than one person.

With diabetes, you're going to need more than one friend, especially in the beginning. I'm not talking about your regular circle of friends and family, although they can bolster you emotionally. The friends I'm talking about are your healthcare professionals, such as your doctor, dentist, and dietitian. There are several others, too, that you'll meet in your journey.

Why do I call them friends? Most of the people in my life whom I consider friends are supportive of my efforts. They like to hear about my plans and successes. They also show understanding when I fall short of expectations—mine or theirs. They give me a good talking to when I need it. They help me understand and learn about new things that I never would have understood without knowing them.

My healthcare friends do the same things for me. They listen when I talk about my illness, applying their knowledge and medical skills to my particular situation. They also have helped me adjust to my new lifestyle. I've had a few stubborn moments about not wanting to change certain patterns. But they got through to me, without being critical or harsh. In talking with them, I have learned ways to manage my illness that I never would have learned on my own.

CREATING YOUR HELP AND HEALTH TEAM

To have the greatest chance of long-term success, here are some of the friendships you need to develop.

Develop a friendship with your primary care physician

A good relationship between you and your primary healthcare provider, such as a general practitioner or an internist, is a powerful tool. Often your primary care doctor makes the diagnosis and provides the basic tools to get you started. Regular appointments with your primary care physician and a certified diabetes educator are some of the best things you can do for yourself in the early weeks.

Once you have been diagnosed with diabetes, your primary care physician should provide a thorough examination. This will include a physical assessment and lots of questions about your health history and current habits. It will probably go something like this:

★ Height and weight measurements

★ Blood pressure check

★ Thyroid examination

★ Examination of hands, fingers, feet, and toes

★ Blood tests for fasting blood sugar, HbA1c, and cholesterol

★ Family history of diabetes, cardiovascular disease, and stroke

★ Prior infections and medical conditions

★ Medications you are taking

★ Smoking history (If you smoke, don't be surprised if your doc strongly encourages you to stop.)

★ Complications with pregnancy or trying to get pregnant

★ Eating and exercise habits

★ Vision abnormalities you may be experiencing

★ Urination abnormalities, which can indicate kidney problems

Make sure your doctor is thorough. Diabetes can be extremely complicated, and your physician needs to have as much information as possible to help you establish a management plan that will work best for you.

Your doctor can also refer you for additional healthcare support. In a large city there may be a diabetes center where several specialists, such as diabetes educators and dietitians, work together as a team. In smaller towns, your healthcare team may come together a little differently, depending on what types of practitioners are in your area. By learning what you need, you can work with your doctor to put together the right group of medical friends.

If you already have a doctor whom you like and trust, you are one step ahead of the game. If you have a doctor but are not sure if he or she is right for you, try the following gut check test: If your doctor was your employee, would you fire her or give her a raise? Answering that question can help determine whether your doctor is right for you. If there is no trust, the relationship can erode quickly. Your health is much too important for you not to have a working relationship based on trust.

If you need to make a change, do so immediately. Ask for referrals from friends, family, and even co-workers. Also, check with your insurance provider to confirm that the physician you chose is covered. If not, you'll have to decide how you will manage the extra costs.

A WORD ABOUT REFERRALS

One of the most important attributes of a good doctor is a willingness to refer. If you have been recently diagnosed with type 2 diabetes, make sure your doctor refers you to an educational program and other specialists as necessary. If your doctor is not willing to make referrals, consider that a big red flag.

Find a good endocrinologist

I liked my primary care doctor. But when I found my endocrinologist, I realized what I had been missing. If you are diagnosed with diabetes, finding an endocrinologist will help you upgrade and fine-tune your diabetes management.

Endocrinologists are trained to understand and treat hormone problems in your system. Recall that insulin is a hormone created by the pancreas. Generally speaking, glands create hormones in small amounts that are then sent into the bloodstream to help regulate many bodily functions, including how well your cells take up the fuel from the food you eat. Besides diabetes, endocrinologists treat other conditions, too, such as thyroid disease and metabolic imbalances.

Ask your primary care doctor to refer you to an endocrinologist or search out someone on your own. You can ask family, friends, colleagues, or people at your diabetes support group. For me, meeting a great endocrinologist helped enormously in understanding and managing my health.

Develop a friendship with a registered dietitian

A registered dietitian (RD) is a professionally trained individual who will focus on your meal planning and weight management goals. A dietitian can also assist you in adapting to your new food goals, such as reducing fat, sodium, or carbohydrate intake (or all three); or reducing calories for weight loss. To find a dietitian, talk with your primary care doctor or other healthcare provider. Your local hospital can also make a referral. Check with your local chapter of the American Diabetes Association, too, to see if they have a list of RDs in your area. Be sure to seek a *registered* dietitian, because he or she has exceptional training and passed a stringent national exam.

HOW A REGISTERED DIETITIAN CAN HELP YOU

The American Diabetes Association has one of the best summaries I've found about how an expert in nutrition helps create an eating plan that works just for you. [9]

Your dietitian helps you figure out your food needs based on your desired weight, lifestyle, medication, and other health goals (such as lowering blood fat levels or blood pressure). Even if you've had diabetes for many years, a visit to the dietitian can help. For one thing, our food needs change as we age. Nutrition guidelines for people with diabetes also change from time to time. Dietitians can also help you learn how:

★ the foods you eat affect your blood sugar and blood fat levels

★ to balance food with medications and activity

★ to read food labels

★ to make a sick day meal plan

★ to plan meals

★ to plan for eating out and special events

★ to include ethnic or foreign foods into your meals

★ to find good cookbooks

★ to make food substitutions

Work with a certified diabetes educator

A certified diabetes educator (CDE) will guide you through the ins and outs of diabetes and provide practical advice. A CDE has undergone extensive professional training, passed a national certification exam, and must be recertified every few years. CDEs are often also nurses, nutritionists, doctors, pharmacists, or others who have a professional healthcare background. Incidentally, CDEs are trained on not only the physical aspects of diabetes but also the psychological facets as well. Often, you'll have three or four in-person visits and then do phone follow-ups. You can also ask them for support and help any time.

WHAT CDEs WANT YOU TO KNOW ABOUT HOW THEY CAN HELP YOU

When it comes to helping people newly diagnosed with diabetes change their lifestyles for better health, Certified Diabetes Educators (CDEs) are advocates, teachers, supporters, and sometimes miracle workers.

Teresa Allen, a registered nurse and a CDE, and Doug Liner, a registered dietitian and CDE, work together in Plano, Texas. Over the years, their dedicated service has resulted in better lives for hundreds of people who have been diagnosed with diabetes. They have some powerful words for you.

Teresa: The biggest change I've seen in the diabetes landscape over the last five to 10 years is that people with diabetes are now more empowered than ever. The person with diabetes is the one who is in control. They should be the top person on the healthcare team, and they are the one making the choices. More and more, that is why places like diabetes education centers exist, because managing diabetes is a tough job. It's not an easy role to take on, and it's too hard to do by yourself. Education centers help patients become the expert on *their* diabetes.

Doug: I agree that patients are more empowered than ever. Second, from the food perspective, carb counting is the focus for controlling blood sugar now, compared to 10 years ago when the focus was often by food group.

Third, from the physician's perspective, there has been advancement in combination therapies—meaning that you might combine lifestyle changes with oral medication to reach your goals.

There's another change, too. I think that the concept of the team approach is coming into its own. We work hard with doctors in the area to let them know that we are a resource for patients who need help in managing diabetes.

Teresa: When you go to your first appointment at a diabetes education center, there are several things you can expect. At our center, for example, we conduct a formal assessment of health. We ask questions about:

★ The foods a patient eats in a day

★ Other medical conditions (hypertension/high cholesterol)

★ Other medications a patient is taking

★ Exercise history

★ Any diabetes maintenance history

★ Glucose monitoring goals

★ A glucose monitor. If a patient does not yet have one, we provide one for them.

Doug: We also set up a carb count on the first visit and talk about the aspects of social dining versus convenience dining versus lazy dining.

Teresa: Generally, we see a patient for three or four in-person visits and then do phone follow-ups. After one year, we send a postcard reminder that we are here for them and can still offer help. Once a person completes our program, we offer support and follow-up for a year at the patient's request.

Doug: Our formal program is 10 hours, done over 45 days. We use those hours flexibly based on our patients' needs. The program includes general instruction, nutritional information, and lifestyle advice. Some instruction is done in a group environment, but there are one-on-one sessions, if necessary. And then we offer the free follow-up care for one year.

Teresa: One of the biggest mistakes I see patients make in the first year of their diabetes management is failing to incorporate exercise into their daily routine. People really seem to fall down on the exercise portion of lifestyle management more than anything.

Doug: You have to own up to this disease, which can be a rough adjustment. One of the biggest challenges that I see patients struggle with is learning when to ask for help. Those who are most successful at managing their disease keep asking questions and keep asking for help when they need it.

Whenever you learn about a new topic, you have to first access the information, then absorb it, integrate it, and own it. If you don't have the desire to ask for help, then you will never get any further along. That's what it comes down to.

Look for a savvy eye doctor (ophthalmologist or optometrist)

Maintaining good control of your blood sugar level is important in helping to preserve your eyesight. Among U.S. adults, diabetes is the primary cause of new cases of blindness. The scary part is that major problems can arise without symptoms, so visit an eye doctor at least once a year for tests. Make sure to bring your eye doctor up to speed on your diabetes, blood sugar history, and the rest of your relevant health history.

Open up to a great dentist

People with diabetes should take meticulous care of their teeth; poorly controlled diabetes can result in serious gum disease and infections, regardless of age. Give your dentist your diabetes background, and listen to his or her recommendations regarding the overall care of your teeth. Depending on your situation, for example, your dentist may suggest you have regular cleanings three times a year, rather than the standard schedule of every six months.

Walk on over to a knowledgeable podiatrist

A podiatrist specializes in treating people with foot problems and performs regular checkups of the feet and toes. People with diabetes may

HIGH BLOOD SUGAR AND
WHITE BLOOD CELLS DON'T MIX

Excess glucose in your blood can wreak havoc on your ability to fight infection. White blood cells defend your body by attacking things like viruses and bacteria that cause infections. But a prolonged level of high blood sugar interferes with white blood cells' ability to kill invading cells. Worse yet, some of the invading cells feed on the extra glucose, thus increasing the chance of infection.

Those with diabetes tend to have more infections: gums, skin, mouth, teeth, feet, genitals, and near an incision site following surgery. If you do get an infection, antibiotics can work wonders. However, long-term use of antibiotics can result in liver damage, so maintaining tight glucose control will go miles in decreasing the chances of developing hard-to-beat infections.

develop poor circulation and nerve problems in the extremities. They can also develop infections. Keep in mind that small sores can quickly cause big problems. If you develop any sore on your foot, get it checked right away.

Count on a cardiologist

High levels of blood sugar do a number on the vessels in your body. That's why heart attacks and strokes are the two biggest causes of death in people with diabetes. Again, keeping blood sugar, blood pressure, and blood cholesterol within normal ranges is vitally important to help prevent future cardiovascular illnesses. If your primary care physician suspects you are at risk of heart disease, he or she will likely refer you to a cardiologist.

For women, talk to your obstetrician/gynecologist

For the women reading this book, did you know that diabetes makes you more prone to yeast infections and urinary tract infections? This is because glucose encourages the growth of yeast in your body. Also note that birth control pills can increase your blood sugar levels, and using them long term may increase the risk of complications. Have checkups on a regular basis so that you and your OB/GYN can see if diabetes is impacting reproductive organs. Your healthcare provider will help you determine how often you should come in for such exams. If you are approaching the end of childbearing years, note that changes in hormonal levels around menopause can lead to higher than normal blood sugar levels. Remember, though, you don't have to do any of this by yourself. Your team is there to support, encourage, and help you manage your health.

A special note to men

Do you need another reason to manage your diabetes well? Poor diabetes control and high blood sugar can lead to erectile dysfunction (ED). Since diabetes affects blood vessels throughout the body, it can eventually damage the vessels and nerves in the penis. Medications or other conditions such as high blood pressure may also lead to ED. So can depression. It's just as important to understand, though, that just because you have diabetes does not mean that you will experience ED. But if you are experiencing problems with erections, see your doctor. Several treatments are available, including oral medications and other types of therapies.

Create a supportive network

Develop a relationship with your local chapter of the American Diabetes Association (ADA). The ADA has fantastic resources to help you learn about and manage your diabetes. The ADA was founded in 1940 with a mission to "prevent and cure diabetes and to improve the lives of all people affected by diabetes." They sponsor community events throughout the nation. To find your local or state chapter, check your phone book. They also have a fabulous Web site at www.diabetes.org, where you can find information about the ADA office closest to you.

Some of your biggest supporters will be your friends and family. There are also diabetes support groups and online chat groups. No matter what your network looks like or how it changes over time, having a cadre of supporters to cheer your successes and hear your frustrations will go a long way in helping you manage this illness. Support can also take the form of talking with a mental health professional. Being diagnosed with diabetes can lead to feelings of failure, frustration, and disappointment. There are many qualified social workers, family therapists, psychologists, and psychiatrists who can assist you in coming to terms with your illness.

DEVELOPING YOUR TYPE 2 ATTITUDE

The best support you can have is a positive and hopeful attitude. Unlike other diseases, with type 2 diabetes, you have a great degree of control. Alterations in lifestyle can make a huge difference in how the disease progresses. Here are some ways to develop your positive outlook:

Develop a friendship with an exercise routine

Exercise is going to be one of your best friends for the rest of your life. Exercise helps bring down your blood sugar by stimulating the muscles to use the glucose that's in your blood. If you are not already exercising regularly, make your initial goal 30 minutes of moderate exercise a day. Brisk walking is perfect for this.

Accept yourself

Some people with type 2 diabetes refuse to accept their situation. Refusal to accept and manage your disease will put you on a path to more serious health problems. So if you have diabetes, accept it and get to work on managing it.

Get smart

There is no shortage of information available to help you manage type 2 diabetes. Learn all you can to best manage your disease. Remember, your healthcare team, your support network, and your friends are pulling for you. They have a lot of information and support to share.

Develop a friendship with your gut instincts

Diabetes management is different for different people. Learn what works best for you. Trust your instincts, take action, and measure your results. One of the biggest challenges is to learn when to ask for help. I quickly learned that the more you ask for help, the better you feel.

CHAPTER 5

THE MIND-BODY CONNECTION

Managing your type 2 diabetes is simple, right? You choose exercise over watching a rerun of *Friends*. You pick lean meats and green vegetables over macaroni and cheese and chocolate éclairs. You figure out ways to lift your mood rather than sink into despair.

Like I said, simple—but not always easy. Shifting into a new attitude may be difficult when you're tossing out old behaviors and inviting new ones in. You're now eating more green foods in a single day than you thought anyone would have ever willingly choked down! Truth be told, I've gotten used to lots of vegetables. I even like them now. During the first few weeks and months, I had to concentrate to choose a side dish of steamed green beans instead of nachos. Sometimes I think my body is finally getting back at me for all those years I didn't listen to my mother when she said, "Eat your vegetables!" Instead, I conspired with the family dog. I snuck those green things off my dinner plate to his waiting muzzle when Mom wasn't looking.

Your daily choices will allow you to make peace with this disease. Choices, though, can be slippery. Even when we know what the right choice is, taking that action can feel like another groaning step up the side of a hard, high, insurmountable mountain. No, our diabetic body does not need a Snickers bar. But our brain tells us that we require that candy bar. And the brain is a formidable force. You need to know how to work with it.

ARE YOU CARRYING BAGGAGE OR A SUITCASE?

The way I see things, we are all taking a particular journey through life, each carrying our own metaphorical suitcase (or baggage, depending on your view of the world). I like the suitcase metaphor because a suitcase is something I can pack and unpack.

I had to decide how to make room for diabetes in my life. If a diabetes diagnosis is part of your life, you will too. Will you cram that diagnosis in your baggage, alongside the lifestyle decisions that probably helped lead to diabetes? Or will you open your suitcase and toss out some of your old ways to make room for this new way of living?

The weight of the luggage you carry has a lot to do with one of the most formidable forces in life: your brain. Brainpower, not brawn, will let you live the best possible life while you manage this illness. When your brain is properly wrapped around diabetes, I guarantee that your body will follow. If you possess the right attitude toward managing your illness, your blood sugar numbers will be in a range that is right for you. If your approach to your revised lifestyle is positive, then the outcome will be positive. Your measurable outcome may be weight loss or a better HbA1c reading. In my experience, the psychological and emotional benefits of actively making daily choices are just as significant as meeting my numerical goals.

Feeling sadness, anxiety, or even depression with this diagnosis is a normal reaction. In fact, at one point after being diagnosed, I burst into tears at work. Yes, I had big feelings and big reactions after being diagnosed, but I was surprised that my usual persona of strength was split down the seams for my office colleagues to see.

That being said, I also firmly believe that attitude and emotions play a huge role in overall health. I have down days about my disease. I've learned to let myself have those feelings, listen to what they're telling me, and then let them go. Sometimes those uncomfortable feelings last a few moments, sometimes they last half a day or even a whole day. But each time they creep up on me, I listen to what they have to say. When they're finished communicating, I'm able to move into a calmer, happier way of looking at the world.

If you have a positive attitude toward the management process, the rest of your diabetes management, should be—well, more manageable. In short, a positive attitude will make your suitcase a whole lot lighter. The American Psychological Association notes, "When people are ill, it's important to deal with the illness on the physical, emotional, and spiritual levels. If you treat just the body, you short-change yourself. We don't know exactly how the mind/body connection works, but we do have biochemical evidence that there's a connection."[10]

Though this book offers some techniques to help keep your spirits up as you adjust to your new lifestyle, it is important to understand that being diagnosed with a serious illness can lead to depression or even posttraumatic stress disorder (PTSD).[11-13] These are serious medical conditions and should not be ignored. If you find yourself anxious, worried, or unable to get through your daily activities, be sure to seek out professional help. There is no shame in asking for assistance. Psychologists, psychiatrists, and counselors work with people every day who are facing life-changing events.

ATTITUDE IS EVERYTHING

I have always been blessed with a positive outlook on things. And when I try to think of how my attitude comes into play, it is not about what has happened to me, but how I react to what has happened. When I was diagnosed, after the initial shock wore off, all I could think was, "Well, it could be worse." And on the scale of chronic illnesses, at least this seemed somewhat manageable.

TURNING A NEGATIVE INTO A POSITIVE

If you don't have a naturally positive outlook on things, how do you get your head turned around to look forward rather than backward? There are many tips and tricks to help you go about this. But in my mind, they all boil down to three basic steps:

1. Recognize negative thoughts or behaviors.

2. Think through an alternate way to address the situation.

3. Put your alternative into practice.

Developing any new habit takes practice. Remember when you took your first blood sugar reading on your own? You were probably a little clumsy. I sure was. But after the tenth time, you had it down. Developing a different outlook is like this, too. Repetition is the key to learning, so as you find methods that work particularly well for you, make sure to use them again and again until they become second nature.

PRACTICE MAKES PERFECT

Here are some techniques that you might try in order to help develop a more positive outlook in managing your diabetes:

Positive mental imagery

For five minutes at night before you drop off to sleep, or for five minutes in the morning before you hop out of bed, imagine what your day would be like as the perfect diabetes manager. See yourself exercising and feel what it is like to exceed a particularly difficult physical goal. Actually feel that emotion. If you wanted to ride your exercise bike for 35 minutes at the "6" setting—something you haven't been able to do yet—picture yourself not only doing that but also feeling proud of yourself. Holding that emotion for as little as 20 seconds helps your body take cues from your brain and understand that you can meet this goal. It might take a few more physical sessions of riding the exercise bike to get your muscles in shape before you meet the goal you've been imagining. But you've set the intention in your mind and held the feeling of success in your body. Your mind, emotions, intention, and muscles will then be working together to meet your goal.

As part of your five-minute daily imagining, also picture yourself at lunch with your colleagues at a restaurant, making healthy choices. Your pals are having burgers, fries, and milkshakes. You're having a fabulous time, listening and chatting while you enjoy your burger with a side salad and a diet soda. Again, feel the emotion of what it's like to make good choices. Feel pride that you were able to pass up that double-chocolate milkshake with extra whipped cream. Again, it's setting the intention and practicing the outcome that lets your brain know that when it's time to order, you're perfectly happy with your burger and salad. Remember, you've seen yourself having a great time. The great time comes from you and your attitude, not the food you eat.

As part of your daily imagery, also feel the satisfaction of taking your blood sugar and getting a reading of, say, 129 mg/dL after eating. Enjoy the contentment of meeting the goal that you've worked so hard to achieve. Your visualization can include a visit to your doctor where you receive unabashed praise for the great job you are doing in controlling the diabetes. Again, feel what it's like to get that kind of praise. Use both your brain and your emotions during your daily five minutes to let your body know what these successes feel like. Your body is getting used to a new way of being, and you need to use your brain and emotions to light the way.

When it comes to positive mental imagery, choose what feels great, and hone in on the details and feelings. Picture the reactions from others as they notice your good work, the aroma that surrounds you as you sit in a café sipping decaf with friends while they eat fattening pastries, or the roar of the crowd as you complete your first 10-kilometer run. The more detailed the imagery, the better it will work.

You might think positive mental imagery is a lot of fluff. Remember though, you are putting new ideas into practice. Give it a try. Many professional athletes, business people, and others use this technique; and many sports psychologists endorse this method. They note that improving execution relies on using all of the senses—sight, smell, hearing, touch. Making the image as visible as possible provides the maximum benefit. When used in addition to physical practice, this technique helps athletes not only enhance learning new skills but also refine performance.

While you may not be a world-class athlete, using positive imagery as part of your diabetes tool kit, practiced over time, can help make your diabetes easier to manage.

Write it down

Often when I am feeling overwhelmed and frustrated, I sit down for a few minutes and write out what I am feeling. (For me, this usually includes several obscenities.) Writing is a simple but powerfully cathartic process. By expelling the gut emotion I am feeling and getting it on paper, I feel relieved of the burden. That process then clears my mind to put things into perspective and helps me determine how to best handle the situation.

I also write down the things that are going right. When I write about a particularly good day, it is something I can reflect on for inspiration and use to remind myself that I am doing things well. Write down positive thoughts about yourself, and reread them often. They will start sticking to your brain like superglue sticks to your fingers.

Surround yourself with positive people

With diabetes, it is critically important for you to identify the people around you who are supportive and understanding of your new challenges. And let me tell you, if you are with people who do not want to take the time to understand what you are going through, it's a drag both emotionally and physically. This doesn't mean you should expect your family and friends to completely rearrange their lives around your diabetes. But I think they should be open to offering you support and listening to your needs. If that is not the case, you may need to make the choice to remove yourself from a situation that is not supportive of or productive for you.

GOAL SETTING

Goal setting is a crucial part of the mind-body connection. When setting your goals in diabetes management (or anything else, for that matter), here are some tips:

Write them down

People who write down their goals typically have a much higher chance of following through on what they have written compared with those who don't.

Be as specific as possible

Goals must be measured, and therefore they need to be defined in a specific, measurable way. Instead of saying your goal is to "lower my blood sugar," say, "For the month of May, I want a daily fasting blood sugar reading of no more than 110 mg/dL." The latter goal can be measured numerically and with a timeline.

Set goals you can control

Create goals that are completely within your control, can be measured, and are realistically achievable. (Remember, when making dieting or exercise goals, always check with your doctor first.) Here are some examples: food intake (I won't have more than a half cup serving of that tiramisu); physical health (I will reduce my body fat measurement by 3 percent over the next three months); and spiritual health (I will volunteer at a food kitchen at least eight hours a month for the next six months).

Develop a plan with benchmarks and write it down

If your goal is to lose 20 pounds over four months, then plan exactly how you will do that. It may involve working out at least five days a week and reducing your caloric intake by 10 percent. Write how you will involve your family and friends. Maybe part of your plan is to put together a lunchtime walking group at work. Set interim goals. If after a month you have lost only one pound instead of the desired five, adjust your plan. Use your written plan to see if you are veering off course.

Reward yourself

Once you achieve your goal, make sure to take some time to congratulate yourself. Reflect on how great it feels to overcome that challenge. Rewards can be small and simple (like a night at the movies with your sweetie) to big and fun (a weekend trip to Las Vegas). I like to keep the reward proportionate to the goal I have achieved. If I meet my workout goals for the month, I treat myself to a new athletic top or new shoes. If I meet my three-month food intake goals, I will treat myself to a two-hour massage. As I write this, my goal is to bring my HbA1c to below 6 percent over the next six months. When I achieve that goal, I guarantee you that a weekend in New York City will be mine. These are rewards that are fun for me. However, I never make the reward about food. It would be just plain counterproductive to celebrate a weight loss goal with a chocolate cake. The key is to find things that are fun for you. You took a lot of time and effort to reach your goal. Don't forget to take the time to reward yourself.

CHAPTER 6

THE SKINNY ON FAT

What if," I wondered as I panted along, trying desperately to finish the 3-mile run, "what if I had trained more and eaten less?" As I imagined myself smugly pushing away that second piece of pie and nobly jumping on the treadmill, runner after runner passed me by. I forced myself to keep moving, my legs feeling like waterlogged wool, my breath fast and shallow. I told myself to be proud I was doing this, to be proud that I finished at all. But it was hard to be proud when I finished dead last.

That race was before I was diagnosed with diabetes. Wondering what might have been didn't help me then, and it doesn't help me now. When I catch myself wondering, "What if I didn't have diabetes?" I quickly bring myself to the here and now. I remind myself that all I have is this moment. And it is in this moment that I can make choices about my life and health.

And some of the most vital choices are centered on diet and exercise. It's not enough to eat a good diet but never get your heart pumping. Conversely, you can exercise every day and still not get the results you want if you don't pay attention to your diet. No matter how much you wish it weren't so, diet and exercise go hand in hand for good diabetes management.

THE "F" WORD

Fat is not a four-letter word. In fact, fat is good. Every person's body requires a minimum amount of fat to function. Fat helps regulate body temperature and provides protective cushioning around our organs. But, like most other things, too little or too much body fat is unhealthy, and you want to stay in a range that is just right. While it's common for many of us to add more body fat as we age, the truth is that increasing age and increasing waistlines don't have to go hand in hand. In fact, what's considered a healthy range of fat remains relatively consistent as we age.

The ideal body fat level is different for women than it is for men. When helping individuals determine where they are on the body fat scale, fitness professionals follow these commonly accepted guidelines:[14]

★ Essential fat: 10–12 percent for women, 2–4 percent for men. This is the minimum level necessary for survival.

★ Athletes: 14–20 percent fat for women, 6–13 percent for men.

★ Fitness: 21–24 percent fat for women, ideally 14–17 percent for men.

★ Acceptable: 25–31 percent fat for women and 18–25 percent for men. Anything above the acceptable level translates into an increased risk of chronic disease.

There are a number of ways to measure body fat, and they range in both price and accuracy. Let's take a look at four of the most popular methods.

Home scales and hand-held devices

Some scales and other devices on the market use bio-electric impedance analysis (BIA) to measure body fat. Impedance in this usage means that a low voltage electrical current is obstructed—impeded—by fat. Fat is a poor conductor of electrical current, so the more fat, the greater the resistance to the current. When done correctly and on properly operating equipment, BIA can yield results that are accurate to within 3 percentage points.[15] But getting an accurate result can be a little tricky sometimes. To get the most accurate measurement, avoid eating and drinking within four hours of the test; avoid exercising within 12 hours; drink no alcohol within 48 hours of the test; and urinate fully prior to the test.

The machines can be expensive, too, ranging from $100 to $400 for individual units. Having a BIA test at a gym or university is less expensive—about $30. Some home scales also have BIA capability built into them, and the cost is a little more reasonable than buying a separate machine. I have one of these scales at home.

As mentioned, the accuracy can be variable. In my case the body fat measurements have been off by as much as 15–20 percent compared to caliper testing done by a certified personal trainer at my local YMCA.

Caliper test

Many of us at some point have had the body fat caliper test, also called a skinfold test. It's both easy and painless. A trained professional measures pinches of fat from several different areas of your body, such as the back of your arm, the front of your thigh, and around your hips and stomach. Those measurements are then mathematically calculated with your height and weight to determine your body fat percentage. Many different types of professionals are trained to perform this test. In most cases (and in my case), the professional is a certified personal trainer. However, it could be a nurse or dietitian or some other medical professional who has this type of training. When performed according to guidelines, this test usually has an accuracy of 3 percent compared to underwater weighing.[15] Costs will vary, but if you are a member of a gym, you can usually get the test done for free or at a discounted rate. If not, other places that perform this test include the YMCA, YWCA, a sports/exercise physiology lab, college, university, or even a wellness program based at a local hospital. If you have trouble finding a place, ask a member of your healthcare team for a referral. Also, make sure the person taking the measurements has at least a year of experience in measuring body fat. Accuracy can vary based on the tester's experience.

BODY FAT MEASUREMENT TIPS FROM A CERTIFIED PERSONAL TRAINER

Marc Mason is certified as both a personal trainer and as a weight management consultant. He's an expert at measuring body fat and in 2007 was named as Kansas City's best personal trainer in *KC Magazine*. When it comes to using calipers to measure body fat, Marc really knows his stuff. He offers some great advice about skinfold testing for those who are new to this technique:

★ Using calipers to measure body fat is a practiced skill, and some people are better at it than others. Caliper aptitude is both an art and a science, like just about everything else in healthcare.

★ Ask how much experience the person conducting your skinfold test has. Experience often translates to greater accuracy. Marc suggests that the person doing your skinfold test have at least 40 to 50 previously supervised measurements.

★ Get your body fat measured every three months to track your progress. If possible, have the same person measure you every time, which again leads to greater accuracy.

★ If you need to lose body fat, be mindful that a goal of reducing your total body fat percentage by 1 to 3 percent every three months is both healthy and achievable for most people. You would want to verify with your doctor a more specific range that is right for you.

Hydrostatic weighing

Hydrostatic weighing is just a fancy term for being weighed under water. In this test, you literally get dunked in a tank of water (exhaling as much as possible before you go under). Because body fat is not dense, people with a higher body fat percentage float higher in the water. In other words, fat floats while muscle and bone do not. This test has a high degree of accuracy, within about 1.5 percent[15] when it is performed within established guidelines. However, accuracy depends somewhat on absolute exhalation before you are dunked. If you have much air in your lungs, it will effect the measurement. This test, which is available at research institutions or universities, can cost anywhere between $25 and $75. If you're not near a local university, ask a member of your healthcare team for a testing location in your area.

You say DEXA, I say DXA

Dual-Energy X-Ray Absorptiometry (DEXA or DXA) is a relatively new technology originally created to measure bone density. Not only does it measure bone mass, it can also determine how much fat you have and where it's located. This test is painless. The whole body is scanned for 10–20 minutes with two low-dose x-rays. Accuracy is typically within 1–3 percent. While highly accurate, it's also a bit pricey, ranging from $100 to $300. This measurement can be performed at hospitals and some physicians' offices, but not all facilities have the proper software to conduct body-fat testing. If you are interested in this body-fat measurement technique, check with your doctor to see if it's available in your area. Depending on your individual circumstances, insurance coverage may help pay for this test.

While it may be hard for you, get your body fat measured and take the steps needed to get yourself into a healthy body-fat range. To paraphrase an old saying, nothing tastes as good as healthy feels.

THE BMI BUZZ

There's a lot of buzz about body mass index (BMI). Body mass index is one way of assessing if a person is overweight or obese. BMI is usually associated with the level of body fat, but unlike the tests mentioned above, BMI does not directly measure it. A high BMI does not necessarily mean excess fat. Some, such as athletes who have a lot of muscle, have a high BMI although they don't have extra fat. Muscle weighs a lot more than fat, so their excess body weight comes from their extra muscle.

BMI is a mathematical calculation that looks at both height and weight. BMI is weight in kilograms divided by height in meters squared (kg/m^2). The table on the next page has done the hard math for you. To estimate your BMI, find your height in the left column. Move across the row to find your weight. The number at the top (19, 20, 21, etc.) is your BMI. Underweight is considered as having a BMI of less than 18.5. Normal weight is a BMI of 18.5–24.9. Overweight is 25–29.9. Obese is a BMI of 30 or greater.

BODY MASS INDEX[16]

BMI (kg/m²)	19	20	21	22	23	24	25	26	27	28	29	30	35	40
Height	Weight (lb.)													
4'10"	91	96	100	105	110	115	119	124	129	134	138	143	167	191
4'11"	94	99	104	109	114	119	124	128	133	138	143	148	173	198
5'	97	102	107	112	118	123	128	133	138	143	148	153	179	204
5'1"	100	106	111	116	122	127	132	137	143	148	153	158	185	211
5'2"	104	109	115	120	126	131	136	142	147	153	158	164	191	218
5'3"	107	113	118	124	130	135	141	146	152	158	163	169	197	225
5'4"	110	116	122	128	134	140	145	151	157	163	169	174	204	232
5'5"	114	120	126	132	138	144	150	156	162	168	174	180	210	240
5'6"	118	124	130	136	142	148	155	161	167	173	179	186	216	247
5'7"	121	127	134	140	146	153	159	166	172	178	185	191	223	255
5'8"	125	131	138	144	151	158	164	171	177	184	190	197	230	262
5'9"	128	135	142	149	155	162	169	176	182	189	196	203	236	270
5'10"	132	139	146	153	160	167	174	181	188	195	202	207	243	278
5'11"	136	143	150	157	165	172	179	186	193	200	208	215	250	286
6'	140	147	154	162	169	177	184	191	199	206	213	221	258	294
6'1"	144	151	159	166	174	182	189	197	204	212	219	227	265	302
6'2"	148	155	163	171	179	186	194	202	210	218	225	233	272	311
6'3"	152	160	168	176	184	192	200	208	216	224	232	240	279	319
6'4"	156	164	172	180	189	197	205	213	221	230	238	246	287	328

Remember that charts such as this one provide only an estimate. If you fall into the overweight or obese category, don't let that discourage or defeat you. *You* define who you are. Use the information only as a starting point. In the next few pages, I'll share what has worked for me. But remember to work with your healthcare team to find a plan, a weight, and a lifestyle that works best for you.

WINNER'S TIPS AND TRICKS

With all of the diets and exercise routines I've tried over the years, one of the most important things I've learned was best expressed centuries ago by a Roman playwright: Moderation in all things.

I recommend that you forget about the extremes and think in terms of moderation. You do not have to lose enough weight to appear in a designer jeans advertisement. You do need to be at a healthy weight that is right for you: a weight that helps keep your blood sugar in check and allows you to feel your best. You do not need to be a world-class athlete, but you do need to incorporate exercise into your daily routine. Just a few minor adjustments to your routine will result in changes that will lead to a longer, healthier life. You can be a hero—to yourself and others who love you and want to keep you around in good health as long as possible.

WHY IS EXERCISE IMPORTANT?

This can be answered in three words: blood sugar control. When you exercise, your muscles are working harder; they need glucose for energy. That's why when you exercise for a sustained amount of time, your blood glucose levels drop. This is not only limited to the time you exercise, but also for hours afterward. Therefore, when you exercise consistently (work out 40–60 minutes a day, six days a week) at a moderate pace, you will likely see better long-term blood sugar readings.

WHAT KIND OF EXERCISE IS BEST FOR ME?

This can be answered in four words: whatever suits you best. No matter what kind of exercise you choose, make sure it is something you enjoy. Walking is a great way to start. It's easy for most of us, can be done with friends or family, and is a great way to get a body moving that has not moved in a while. Notice I said walking. Not sauntering or strolling, and not speeding to the point you are breathless. Moderation.

If your exercise routine for the last several years has consisted of shuffling from the couch to the refrigerator and back, don't worry. You're going to do just fine. Set a goal of walking around the block. Maybe two blocks. Tomorrow, go half a block farther. The day after tomorrow, go another half a block. Remember: Just walk a bit farther tomorrow than you did today. Do that for each of your tomorrows, and you'll be surprised at how fast you'll work up to half a mile. Then three-quarters of a mile. Then a mile. Yes, a mile. I bet you won't stop at a mile. As your muscles start to wake up, they're going to want to get moving and keep moving. In a matter of just a couple of weeks, instead of dreading your walk, you're going to look forward to it—and your muscles won't be able to wait. They'll look forward to how good they feel. I'll also bet that you're going to want to start moving faster, too. Simply listen to and follow your body's cues. If you went eight blocks today and want to go nine tomorrow in the same amount of time, give it a try. If you get too winded, your body will tell you to slow down. Remember, always listen to and heed your body's signals. A little extra effort to get air into your lungs is good when you exercise. Gasping for air and clutching your side is not.

WHAT ARE MY EXERCISE OPTIONS?

One word: limitless. You can walk, ride a bike, mountain climb, join a gym, swim, or do whatever gets your body moving. Weight training can be especially good because the more muscle you have, the more glucose you burn. If the thought of weight training right now sounds out of reach, don't worry. You can work up to it in time. If you don't want to exercise alone, engage a friend, your kids, your spouse, or even recruit the pooch. Fido will probably enliven your walks with canine antics and a friendly wag at passersby.

If an outdoor activity is your exercise of choice, have a backup plan for bad-weather days. Go to the mall and walk inside for half an hour or longer. Buy a treadmill or an elliptical trainer. I use an elliptical trainer on the days I can't get out. I love it because I can still watch TV while actually doing something good for my body and my mood. Exercise is one of the best ways to lift your spirits if you're feeling down. Here are some other options to help you fit exercise into your daily routine:

★ Take the stairs instead of the elevator.

★ If you take the bus or city train, get off one stop early and walk the last block or two to your home or office.

★ Going grocery shopping today? Before you grab your cart, walk the inside perimeter of the store five times.

★ Walk a little more briskly at the mall. And skip the greasy snacks at the food court.

★ Take pride in parking in the spot farthest away from the door. You will get in more walking. The added bonus is that you'll probably avoid door dings.

★ Ride a bike, and don't forget it's fun!

You can also think about joining the gym. Gyms offer a variety of exercise options—treadmills, elliptical trainers, stationary bikes, rowing machines, aerobics classes, Pilates workouts, and maybe even belly dancing or kickboxing.

EXERCISE ALERT

If injury, disability, or excessive weight won't allow you to walk, work closely with your physician to come up with a plan that will let you move to the best of your ability. If you cannot walk, think about the possibility of using water to exercise: Swimming, water aerobics, and water therapy are just some examples. Note, too, that many YMCAs with swimming pools have a chairlift system to help people who are unable to use the steps get in and out of the water.

FOOD AS FUEL

Much like exercise is an individual experience, finding a good eating plan that's just right for you will take some time and tinkering.

If you go through any kind of formal diabetes education, chances are you have been exposed to the diabetic diet. This way of eating is reasonable and works for many people with diabetes. I followed the plan myself for six months or so and found it similar to the Weight Watchers approach. The diet is based on exchanges. For example, at a meal you might have one carbohydrate exchange and one protein exchange. However, I still felt hungry a lot of the time, so I began to tinker. Now, after managing my illness for a few years, I feel I am in good control of my diet. (Perfect control? No. Good control? Yes.) Through experimentation, close monitoring of my blood sugar, and my own gut feel, I have a daily routine that leaves me satisfied food-wise and with blood sugar in control. I won't go into the specifics of exactly what I eat, because what works for me may not work for you. The point is to try new things, see how it impacts your blood sugar control (remember to measure, measure, measure), and find what works best for you.

THE GLYCEMIC INDEX

In recent years, there's been a lot of discussion about the glycemic index (GI). Books and Web sites are devoted to the topic, and all sorts of articles have been published about it in the popular press and medical literature. Though the glycemic index has been around for more than 20 years and has been refined over time, some experts say that there's not enough evidence to show that trading high-glycemic foods for solely low-glycemic foods will improve blood sugar control. They argue that eating only low GI foods does not necessarily make for a healthy diet. Their recommendation is to choose a nutritionally balanced diet while controlling overall carbohydrates. If your blood sugar levels are high after consuming certain foods, they advise you to eat less of those particular foods or adjust mealtime medication.[17]

I turned to the glycemic index at first to help me understand what might spike my blood sugar. But I have never solely relied on it or any other single diet in my eating plan. I learned how to manage my blood sugar by measuring, measuring, measuring and taking advice from my own healthcare team.

Because you'll probably run across it as you learn the ins and outs of managing your blood sugar, here's a quick overview of the glycemic index.

The glycemic index is simply a scale. It ranks food by how fast it can raise your blood sugar level, as compared to a reference food. The reference food is either white bread or glucose. Recall that carbohydrates break down during digestion, and it's glucose from those carbs that provide energy for your body to function. The blood sugar increase after you eat is called the glycemic response. The glycemic response is influenced by a lot of things, including how much you eat and whether the food is heavily or lightly processed.

The glycemic index ranges from 1 to 100. In general, low glycemic index foods have a value of 55 or less (for example, kidney beans), medium glycemic index foods range from 56 to 69 (such as an orange), and high glycemic index foods are those with a value of 70 or more (regular soda, for instance).

There's another measure that you'll likely run across. It's the glycemic load (GL) and is often seen along with the glycemic index. The glycemic index compares foods containing equal amounts of carbohydrates. But in real life, we don't eat that way. We eat big portions, little portions, bite-sized things, and sometimes tub-sized things (like those tubs of popcorn I used to eat at movies). The glycemic load, which also is a scale from 1 to 100, is calculated from the food's specific glycemic index value, the serving size, and the amount of carbohydrates in a serving. The higher the glycemic load, the higher the expected rise in blood glucose.

The glycemic index and glycemic load may serve as guidelines for selecting foods to incorporate or avoid as part of your eating plan. However, it's still important to work with your physician, CDE, or registered dietitian to establish a meal plan that is right for you. Only through careful blood glucose monitoring and working with your healthcare team can you best determine what effects certain foods will have on you and your diabetes management goals.

GLYCEMIC INDEX AND GLYCEMIC LOAD
VALUES OF SELECTED FOODS[18]

FOOD	GLYCEMIC INDEX (white bread=100)	SERVING SIZE (grams)	GLYCEMIC LOAD PER SERVING
Bakery Products			
Banana cake, made with sugar	67	80	18
Chocolate cake, made from packet mix, with frosting	54	111	20
Bran muffin	85 ± 8	57	15
Pastry	84	57	15
Beverages			
Cola	90	250 mL	16
Smoothie, soy/banana	43	250 mL	7
Apple juice, pure, cloudy, unsweetened	53	250 mL	10
Orange juice, unsweetened, reconstituted	79	–	–
Breads			
Bagel, white frozen	103 ± 5	70	25
Oat bran bread, 50%	63 ± 10	30	8
Cracked wheat kernel bread, 50%	84 ± 4	30	12
White flour bread	100	30	10
Cereal Grains			
Pearl barley	32 ± 3	–	–
White rice, boiled	99	150	30
Brown rice, steamed	72	150	16
Parboiled rice	103	150	26
Bulgur wheat, boiled 20 min.	65 ± 4	–	–
Dairy Products and Alternatives			
Ice cream, premium chocolate	53	50	4
Milk, full fat	57	–	–
Low-fat yogurt, fruit, aspartame	20	200	2
Low-fat yogurt, fruit, sugar	47	200	10
Soy milk	63	250	8

FOOD	GLYCEMIC INDEX (white bread=100)	SERVING SIZE (grams)	GLYCEMIC LOAD PER SERVING
Fruit			
Apple	57	120	6
Apricots, dried	43	60	8
Mango	59	120	8
Orange	69 ± 11	120	5
Peach	40	120	4
Pear, Bartlett	58 ± 7	120	3
Plum, raw	23	120	3
Legumes and Nuts			
Chickpeas, dried, boiled	44 ± 8	150	9
Kidney beans	33	150	6
Lentils, red, dried, boiled	25	150	3
Peas, dried, boiled	32	150	2
Snack Foods			
Corn chips, plain, salted	60 ± 5	50	11
Fruit bar, apricot filled	71	50	17
Life Savers, peppermint	100	30	21
M&Ms, peanut	47	30	6
Peanuts	19	50	1
Popcorn, plain, cooked in microwave	79	20	6
Vegetables			
Carrots	131	80	5
Green peas, frozen, boiled	55	80	3
Potato, russet, baked without fat, 45-60 min.	112	–	–
Sweet corn, boiled	85	80	11

This sample shows only a handful of the hundreds of foods whose glycemic index and glycemic loads have been estimated. The first column with numbers shows the food's glycemic index compared to the reference food (in this case, white bread). The higher the number, the higher the glycemic index. The next column shows the quantity of food used to calculate the glycemic load. The final column contains the glycemic load value. Again, the bigger the glycemic load value, the greater impact on blood sugar. Note that the glycemic index and glycemic load of foods vary greatly depending on brand and processing, how the food is cooked at home, and even where the food is grown.

PORTION CONTROL

For me, portion control was—and is—the hardest part of having diabetes. Most of us today, myself included, suffer from portion distortion. We think the mound of food in front of us is one serving. Most of the time it's probably two or three servings.

I have to constantly remind myself that there's a difference between a serving and a shovelful. When I began to use a small kitchen scale to weigh out my food, I was surprised to learn what three ounces of chicken actually looked like. I used the scale for about four months, and quickly learned to eyeball my way to better portion control. I learned that a serving size of protein is equivalent to the size of the palm of your hand. A serving of vegetables or carbohydrates would be about fist-size. The American Dietetic Association offers excellent comparisons to help you visualize portion size:[19]

★ A teaspoon of margarine is the size of the tip of your thumb to the first joint.

★ Three ounces of meat is the size of a deck of cards.

★ One cup of pasta is the size of a tennis ball.

★ One half of a medium bagel is the size of a hockey puck.

★ An ounce and a half of cheese is the size of three dominoes.

★ Two tablespoons of peanut butter are the size of a ping pong ball.

★ One-half cup of vegetables is the size of a light bulb.

Also, be careful when you order food at restaurants. Restaurants love to pile on the portions. At restaurants I only eat half of what is served (except a salad with light dressing). That way my portions are in control, and I have lunch for the next day. It's like getting two meals for the price of one. I've even eaten with friends who tell the waiter to box up half the meal before it arrives at our table. Our dinner arrives at the table, along with a ready-to-go doggy bag. It's a good trick.

A NOTE ABOUT WINES

While most doctors and other health professionals will advise you to keep your alcohol intake to a minimum, it is possible to enjoy wine and spirits—in moderation—as part of your overall healthy diet. When counting calories and carbohydrates, here are a few things to keep in mind when choosing wine.

★ Discuss your alcohol consumption with your healthcare team. They will be able to give you the best individualized advice, especially as it pertains to mixing alcohol with the medications you may be taking.

★ The drier the wine, the less residual sugar it contains. Residual sugar is the natural sugar found in wine after the fermentation process.

★ Dry wines are those that do not have sugar added after the fermentation process.

★ A serving of wine is typically 4 ounces, but a typical restaurant pour is 6 ounces. This is good to keep in mind when counting calories.

★ Dessert wines, such as port, tend to have the highest amounts of sugar content.

★ For some people, alcohol may lower blood sugar; and for others, alcohol raises blood sugar. If you choose to consume alcohol, keep your blood glucose meter close by, and carefully monitor your blood sugar.

ELIMINATE THE NOTION OF DIETING

Your diet is what you consume. Once you unchain yourself from the popular concept of being on a diet you are free to be flexible with a healthy eating plan. Create an eating plan you can live with and enjoy—one that fills your stomach as well as your mind, body, and spirit.

PUTTING IT ALL TOGETHER

As I mentioned earlier, your food plan and exercise routine work best when they work together. There are three steps I encourage you to follow:

1. Plan ahead

On Sunday night, grab your calendar and take about 15 minutes to plan the week. Plan your exercise schedule. Before work or after? Forty minutes or an hour, and on what equipment? Write it down. Then think about your meal planning. Do you have any business dinners where it will be easy to overindulge? What will you do in that situation? How will you plan to make the right decisions when the time comes? By taking the time to think and plan ahead, your opportunity for success is far greater.

2. Think before you act

How many times have you sat down to a meal and just devoured it without thinking? Were you even all that hungry? What do you need to get from each meal? Do you think of eating as nutritional recharge or simply a festival for the taste buds? By just taking 30–60 seconds before a meal and thinking things through, you can plan what you need to accomplish. For example, before demolishing that hamburger and fries, consider eating only half the bread and half the fries. You still get the great taste, but with less of a blood sugar spike and several hundred less calories. If you know you're going to eat a piece of your friend's world-famous cake for dessert, think ahead and skip the bread that she serves with the entrée.

This process does not take long, but it does take a bit of getting used to. Write yourself a note and place it by your dinner plate. Or tell your family to help remind you to think for a few moments before the first forkful goes into your mouth. By taking this one small step, you are setting yourself up for future success.

One of the habits I broke by using this method was eating before bedtime. I would eat right before bed, not because I was hungry, but simply because it was part of my routine. I have significantly curbed this unhealthy habit by asking myself, "Am I really hungry?" and "How will this affect my blood sugar?"

3. Write it down

It is rewarding to see your accomplishments over time. In the same calendar where you wrote your plan, make comments about meeting your goals and how that felt. I love to ride my bike for exercise, and my mileage has been increasing steadily over time. I always keep track of my exercise, because I feel great when I see that three months ago I was averaging 50 miles a week, and now I average 100. I would never know this feeling if I did not write it down.

A LESSON FROM MASTER YODA

One of my favorite movie scenes comes from *The Empire Strikes Back*. Master Yoda is teaching young Luke Skywalker about how to use his inherent power to move heavy objects. Luke struggles mightily and finally lifts a rock or two. Yoda then challenges his protégé to lift the sunken X-wing fighter out of the swamp. Luke tries and fails. In childish frustration, he tells Yoda the task is too big. Without missing a beat, Master Yoda says, "You must unlearn what you have learned….Try not. Do. Or do not. There is no try."[20] Master Yoda then uses his significant powers of both mind and understanding to lift the huge craft out of the water.

Shifting your ingrained attitudes about eating and exercise may at first feel like moving an X-wing fighter out of the murky depths. But when it comes to only trying to manage your disease, I'm in complete agreement with Master Yoda: There is no try. There is only do.

CHAPTER 7

TRACK YOUR PROGRESS

You're dedicated to taking your medication. You're vigilant about your diet. You exercise six days a week. Your diabetes is under control, right? Not necessarily. Even with all of your good work, your blood sugar level can have big swings during the day. Think of one of those beautiful old carousel rides you see at fairs. The horses go up and down all day long. That's what your blood sugar does all day, too. How high and how low it goes depends on what you eat, how much exercise you get, how much diabetes medication you take, how much stress you're under, and whether you're sick with a cold or the flu or another more serious illness.

Everyone's body reacts differently to foods, exercise, stress, and illness. Monitoring your blood sugar levels will let you find how each of these factors affects you. Monitoring will also let you make your own decisions about how to manage your illness.

Making daily notations in your logbook is crucial during the first few months as you establish new behavior patterns toward food and exercise.

This chapter will cover the importance of a diabetic action plan, including the following:

★ Why we need to measure (it's solid proof that we're making progress, and it shows how well we're following our action plan)

★ What to measure (blood sugar, HbA1c, and weight)

★ When to measure

WHY DO WE MEASURE?

We measure to track our progress and make sure we are moving toward our goals. Can you imagine having a goal of saving up an extra $1,000 over a year's time and never checking your account balance to see your progress? With diabetes tracking, our daily progress is hugely important. First, we can learn if we are managing in the right way; and second, we can show our measurements to our healthcare team and work with them to make adjustments if necessary.

Now, to be perfectly honest, I wasn't very thorough when it came to measuring things after I was first diagnosed. I would take my blood sugar, write it down in a little book that came with my blood glucose monitor, and then take that book to my doctor at my checkups. I did it because that's what I was told to do. The problem, however, was that the numbers had no relevance to me other than being high or low. I wasn't using the numbers to see if I was making progress.

My doctor would see a book of numbers, and after a quick glance he would tell me if they were high or low. I have since learned how important tracking my blood sugar level is in helping me reach my goals.

WHAT AND WHEN DO WE MEASURE?

The primary aspect of diabetes management is measuring your blood sugar and then making adjustments in diet, medication, or activity levels if the blood sugar is too high or too low. In the first few months of measuring, you will want to measure more often, because you will want to see how your blood sugar reacts to the foods you eat and your exercise plan.

As you learn your body's patterns, you may be able to measure less often. Remember, blood sugar levels change throughout the day, and a blood sugar measurement reflects that specific moment in time.

At a minimum, you should measure your fasting blood sugar and take another blood sugar measurement at least once again during the day. I measure mine several times each day, but work with your doctor to see how often is right for you.

Second, you will want to track your daily carbohydrate intake. I try to keep my total carbohydrate intake between 75–100 grams per day. My doctor suggested that level, and it seems to work well for me. Work with your healthcare team to find what's right for you. Remember, carbohydrate consumption will directly impact your blood sugar levels.

Third, track your HbA1c levels. I keep a separate sheet of paper in my desk to track my HbA1c progress. I go to the doctor and have an HbA1c test about every three months, so I can see how I have managed my diabetes over that period of time.

I still tend to keep track of my blood sugar and HbA1c levels on paper. I just find that with my life and lifestyle, it works well for me. However, I advocate each person using what works for them. If you prefer to track on the computer, then do it. Many blood glucose monitors have adapters that plug into your computer and upload information. Or just use a simple spreadsheet. The point is to consistently track your blood sugar levels in whatever way works best for you.

Lastly, if you're overweight, track your weight loss. I recommend buying a digital scale and weighing yourself once a week. From a consistency standpoint, I weigh myself on Sunday mornings before breakfast. If you have gained a couple of pounds over the week, make an immediate course correction by adding in more exercise or making better food choices. I know from experience, the more extra weight you carry, the harder it is to manage your diabetes.

I do believe that even people who are not overweight need to keep a close eye on their weight. There are a couple of reasons for this. First, a normal, healthy weight is best to keep your body working at peak performance. Second, by watching weight changes closely, you can make course corrections earlier. It is much easier to lose three pounds than 15. Third, depending on medications you are taking, you could experience weight gain or loss. You should carefully note these changes and report them to your healthcare team, as they could be indicators of other health changes that are taking place. Having said all this, there is a difference between closely watching your weight and being obsessed by it. Know where that line is, and try not to cross it.

TRACKING YOUR PROGRESS

I have developed my own system for tracking my diabetes progress. It is simple to do, does not take much time, and is easy for a doctor to look at and analyze.

I couldn't find the kind of charts I needed, so I ended up creating my own. I made two. The first I use exclusively to track my fasting blood sugar. On the second chart, I record all other aspects of my daily diabetes management activities.

Let's talk about the fasting blood sugar chart first. With this chart both you and your doctor can know if you are in the correct ideal daily fasting blood sugar range. On the chart, you plot your fasting blood sugar against a particular day.

Fasting blood sugar measurements are important for a couple of reasons. First, it is typically the only measurement of the day where you will get a blood sugar reading after having nothing to eat or drink for at least eight hours. Since there are clear recommendations from diabetes experts as to what a healthy range of fasting blood sugar is, you can use these measurements to track how well you're doing on your management plan. Second, you want to check fasting blood sugar to ensure your blood sugar is not too low, since you have not (typically) eaten overnight. If my fasting blood sugar is under 70 mg/dL, I eat 15 grams of a simple carbohydrate immediately, then wait 15 minutes and measure again to see if my blood sugar has returned to a healthy range. If not, then I eat another 15 grams of simple carbs, and measure again in 15 minutes. If you experience hypoglycemia and at any time feel faint or dizzy, call for medical help immediately.

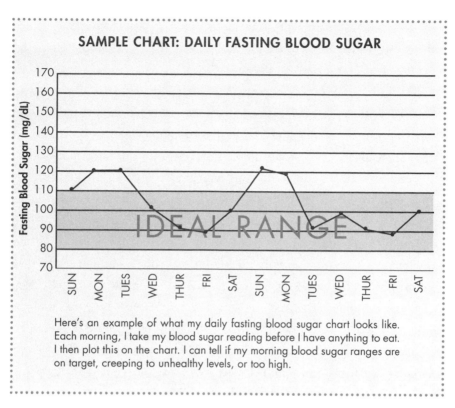

SAMPLE CHART: DAILY FASTING BLOOD SUGAR

IDEAL RANGE

Here's an example of what my daily fasting blood sugar chart looks like. Each morning, I take my blood sugar reading before I have anything to eat. I then plot this on the chart. I can tell if my morning blood sugar ranges are on target, creeping to unhealthy levels, or too high.

The American College of Endocrinology, a highly respected organization of physicians who treat diabetes and other endocrine gland disorders, calls for keeping fasting blood sugar at 110 mg/dL or less.[7] With this general range in mind, I've come up with my own system that helps me know I'm managing my daily blood sugar fluctuations so my pre-meal morning blood sugar levels stay where they're supposed to.

★ 80–110 mg/dL: Right on!

★ 110–130 mg/dL: A little high. What changes can I make to bring these measurements down 10–20 percent?

★ Above 130 mg/dL: Too high. I need to work with my healthcare team to bring these numbers into a healthier range.

This system is beautifully simple. At one glance I can see whether my fasting blood sugar level is within the recommended guidelines. I work hard to keep my morning fasting blood sugar in a healthy zone. If my fasting blood glucose is too high, I take steps *that day*—reducing carbs and/or increasing exercise—to bring it down.

If your fasting blood sugar is too high, you can do small things immediately that pay off big. First, if you are taking diabetes medication, make sure you are taking it exactly as your doctor has prescribed. Also, to bring blood sugar down, you can take a nice 30-minute walk, or any other moderate activity. Cut down on your refined carbohydrate intake. Having a sandwich for lunch? Eat only half the bread, and choose a green salad instead of fries. Small changes can quickly make a big difference.

Having said that, diabetes is a marathon rather than a sprint. While you can make choices that will quickly impact your blood sugar, the end goal is to maintain blood sugar readings that are in a consistently healthy range over the long term. Keeping your blood sugar tightly within a range of 100–130 mg/dL is far healthier than bouncing up and down in a range of 75–200 mg/dL. Consistently healthy blood sugar ranges are derived from making consistently good choices when it comes to balancing eating, exercise, positive attitude, and for most of us, medication.

The second chart allows me to write down what I eat, my carbohydrate intake, my exercise program, blood sugar measurements, and at what time all this occurs. This allows me to see the relationship between food intake, exercise, and my blood sugar. Look at the chart on the next page to see what I mean.

DAILY FOOD, BLOOD SUGAR, AND ACTIVITY LOG

TIME	FOOD	CARBS	BLOOD SUGAR (mg/dL)	EXERCISE
6:00 a.m.	2 cups black coffee		107 (fasting)	
6:30 a.m.				
7:00 a.m.				
7:30 a.m.				
8:00 a.m.	Breakfast—peanut butter on wheat toast	15		
8:30 a.m.				
9:00 a.m.			130	
9:30 a.m.				
10:00 a.m.	Snack—low-fat yogurt and apple	30		
10:30 a.m.				
11:00 a.m.			115	
11:30 a.m.				
12:00 p.m.				
12:30 p.m.	Lunch—chicken Caesar salad, diet soda. Choc. chip cookie	15 40		
1:00 p.m.				
1:30 p.m.				
2:00 p.m.			170	
2:30 p.m.				
3:00 p.m.	Snack—1/4 cup almonds, banana	30		
3:30 p.m.				
4:00 p.m.				
4:30 p.m.				45 min. bike ride

TIME	FOOD	CARBS	BLOOD SUGAR (mg/dL)	EXERCISE
5:00 p.m.				
5:30 p.m.			72	
6:00 p.m.	Dinner—vegetable soup, pork chop, mixed veggies, 1 cup low-fat yogurt	40		
6:30 p.m.				
7:00 p.m.				
7:30 p.m.				
8:00 p.m.			150	
8:30 p.m.				
9:00 p.m.				
9:30 p.m.				
10:00 p.m.			130 (bedtime)	
10:30 p.m.				
11:00 p.m.				
Total		170		

Notes: Good workout today. Next lunch—skip the cookie!

I can do a quick bit of math to see the carbohydrate count for that day was 170 grams. The cookie I ate at lunch caused my blood sugar to shoot up to 170 mg/dL. Yikes. However, check out my blood sugar after exercising: 72 mg/dL. That's cutting it a little too close to hypoglycemia (low blood sugar), which is 70 mg/dL or lower. My blood sugar dropped to a range that I was uncomfortable with, even though I had no symptoms of hypoglycemia. I immediately ate something to make a correction. That is why it is so important to check blood sugar often, so you can head off potential problems before they get too serious.

It's helpful to use these charts and journals every day. The key is to learn how to chart your behavior; see the relationship between food, exercise, and blood sugar; and follow what works best for you. In Appendix 2, you'll find several blank charts to get you started. Feel free to make copies as you need to. I keep my charts in a three-ring binder so my information is quickly at hand.

Seeing your daily progress is a fantastic way to see the results of all your hard work. Keep it up!

CHAPTER 8

DIABETES IN THE EVERYDAY WORLD

W hen it comes to sharing the news, remember that it's entirely up to you who in your life gets to know that you have diabetes. However, I do think it's important to tell those closest to you. The people who love you can anchor you when you're emotionally adrift, shore you up when you're sinking, and cheer you on as you achieve your goals.

I told my family almost right away. At the time, I lived in Seattle and they lived in the Midwest. When I got the news, no distance was too far for me to leave them out of this. We've always been close, and I knew they would help me adjust simply by giving me their love and humor. Thanksgiving was the first major holiday after my diagnosis, and I knew that particular dinner was going to be a challenge. My family, of course, knew I had diabetes; but they had never experienced what that meant. I had always embraced the holidays, blissfully piling my plate with everything. Though I looked forward to my first trip home after the diagnosis, I was nervous about handling the dinner-table temptations.

My family turned that first holiday into loads of laughs. They were respectful, helpful, amusing, and loving as they made light-hearted fun of my new way of eating. It took willpower to get through that first holiday meal on just turkey, salad, vegetables, and one cranberry muffin (instead of my usual three). Their support and banter helped keep me on track and got me through my first major holiday.

AT WORK

Medical information is confidential. However, I do think that it's important to let at least some people at work know. Once you tell them, you have potentially enlarged your network of supporters.

Though I talked to my family nearly right away, I did not immediately tell my co-workers. Initially, I wanted to keep my new health status private. I knew I would tell them, eventually, but I hadn't quite found the right time. For weeks, I soldiered on. At work, I'm usually known as strong, even intimidating, when I need to be. But after I was diagnosed, I knew, deep down, that an emotional storm was brewing.

About a month after my doctor said I had diabetes, I was in my office when a colleague came in to complain about a minor matter. For some reason, my co-worker's little grievance tipped the scale. I started bawling, breaking my hard-and-fast rule to never cry at work. Unfortunately, letting loose wasn't a private affair. My office had three glass walls; everyone nearby could see something was up. Another colleague stepped in to find out what was wrong. He took one look at the tears streaming down my face and scooted out. I calmed myself and a few minutes later walked into his office. I told him that I had been diagnosed with diabetes about a month earlier and that it just all caught up with me.

Ironically, the second colleague also had type 2 diabetes (which was well known at the company), so he could identify with what I was going through. The bright side of my story is that people at work were supportive once they knew. If I needed to take a break to get something to eat, there was no question about it. Most importantly, I still did my job, every day, just like before my diagnosis.

My way of telling people at work turned out to be a little rocky. Yours doesn't have to be. Regardless of whom you tell and how you say it, understand that managing your diabetes at work is similar to managing your diabetes in other parts of your life. You work it in. You have your blood glucose monitor handy and use it. You follow your eating schedule, just as you would if you were not at work. Many days I had back-to-back meetings, so I was always prepared with a protein bar in case I got hungry. I also used my lunch breaks for power walks. That helped my body and cleared my mind. During the summer, I would get a group of people together for a 30-minute walk during lunch time or after work.

Whether or not you tell your workmates is up to you. But if you do decide to keep your situation private, you might consider at least telling a member of the human resources team about your diabetes. They will keep the information confidential, and should you encounter a medical emergency that leaves you unable to talk, that HR person will know to communicate your situation to medical personnel.

A FEW WORDS ABOUT INSURANCE

My insurance coverage has run the gamut. It's ranged from great employer-sponsored coverage to minimal individual coverage. The biggest challenge of all, though, was having no prescription drug coverage. During those months, I was spending in excess of $1,000 per month to pay for medications. I was literally pushing off car repairs and other items to make sure I could pay for the medicine I needed. That was hardly an ideal situation. But my bottom-line commitment was to my health, so I had to make some difficult choices about what to juggle to stay healthy. I hope you won't ever find yourself in that kind of situation. If you do, though, I encourage you to examine what's most important to you (which I hope is your health), and make smart choices based on that commitment. As you learn about your insurance coverage, it may help to keep the following points in mind.

Ask lots of questions

Insurance coverage varies greatly from company to company, and from state to state. For example, a state may require insurance companies and health maintenance organizations that provide group policies to cover certain diabetes-related services, equipment, and supplies. But this legal requirement might not apply to individual policies, self-insured employers, or self-insured union plans, for example. Start asking your insurance company lots of questions after you're diagnosed. That's what customer representatives are there for—to help you understand your benefits.

Know what's covered

Some insurance providers help pay for the cost of blood glucose monitor test strips. However, you can't get the discounted price unless your healthcare provider writes you a prescription. This can be confusing, since test strips can be bought over the counter without a prescription. Again, ask your insurance provider what items (or services) are covered with a written prescription or referral, if needed.

Develop good R_x sense

Under some insurance plans, you can save money by ordering your prescription medications through a mail-order pharmacy. What does your plan offer?

If needed, inquire about prescription assistance

Most pharmaceutical companies offer assistance to people who need help in affording medications and meet a list of qualifying criteria.

Compare plans

If you purchase individual coverage, be diligent in comparing different plans. I have found obtaining a strong insurance plan as an individual is extremely challenging. In my experience, most insurance companies will not provide exceptional coverage unless dictated by state law.

Learn about the high-risk pool

Currently, 30 states have programs to assist people who might be considered uninsurable by private insurance companies due to health conditions. Depending on your situation, you may qualify for limited benefits. To see a list of the states that participate in this program, visit the American Diabetes Association (ADA) site at www.diabetes.org and type "high risk pool" into the site's search box.

FAMILY DEMANDS

Diabetes is a disease that needs a schedule. If you're going to manage it well, then you need to create a schedule that works for you and the others in your household. If going to the gym right after you leave the office is the best time for you, then someone else may have to handle dinner duty. Or if you're an early riser and exercising first thing in the morning is best, you'll probably have to negotiate who feeds the kids, packs the school lunches, and takes them to the bus stop while you're in the gym.

Maybe it's just you and your partner. Even though there are fewer schedules to juggle, fitting diabetes care into the daily scheme of things can still take work. If you and your significant other are used to eating at a certain time—say later in the evening after you get home from a long day in the office—you may have to adjust your mealtime. You may end up eating a bit of dinner at the office to keep your blood sugar levels stable instead of coming home ravenous and eating a big meal with your sweetie.

Maybe your significant other is a gourmet cook and is used to creating lavish meals for both of you to share and enjoy. If those epicurean foods involve high sugar, high carbohydrates, and high fat, your gourmet cook will have to start adding different fare to the repertoire. Don't mistake what I'm saying. You won't have to go on a Spartan diet. You will, however, have to adjust what you eat, when you eat, and how much you eat to help bring your blood sugar levels within healthier ranges.

FAMILY TACTICS

There are several things you can do to help your family understand how important these changes are. Hold a family meeting. Explain what diabetes is. Talk about how important exercise and different food choices are in your life. If your family is used to picking up a drive-through dinner a couple of nights a week after soccer or ballet practice, let them know that this will probably have to stop—especially if it's hard for you to say no to a burger, large fries, and chocolate shake.

When you talk with the kids, don't be surprised if they put up some resistance about this new way of eating. Explain that this is not some fad diet. Get their thoughts about foods they want to eat that you can eat too. As you talk, write down the healthy foods they say they'll eat. Serve one or more of those foods the next time you cook dinner. Then add one or two new healthy foods into each week's meals. If the kids tell you that the new, healthy food you just served is especially yummy, add it to your permanent list. Keep going like this for a few weeks. Within just a couple of months, you're going to have a list of new foods that your whole family will enjoy. Don't be afraid to experiment and add to the list. Refer to it if you're stymied about how to keep food choices interesting over time.

Involve your family and be an example for them. Don't just tell them what to do, show them. Show them you have a good attitude about changing for the better. Show them how to pass up fast food. Take the kids outside for a walk in the park. Reward healthy behavior. Set the example and ultimately your kids will follow you into good health habits.

There's another list to consider keeping, especially in the first few weeks and months. And that's a running list of questions. Not just your questions, but your family's questions, too. Next time you see your doctor, take these questions with you. Think about taking a family member with you, too, so he or she can see exactly what happens when you go for your regular checkups.

You're not the only one who can benefit from taking a diabetes education class. Members of your family can take them too, or go with you to yours. The more information they have, the more they will be able to help you. There's an even bigger benefit, too. Since diabetes runs in the family, there's a chance your children could develop it later in life. The more they know now about food and lifestyle choices that could help prevent diabetes later on, the better off they'll be.

I'd like to add a special note to women. In the last few decades, we've come a long way from being the ones who solely handle all of the tasks that keep daily life running smoothly. But the truth is that women still perform the largest chunk of family and household management. Life is busy with working, doing household chores, carving out quality time with the kids, and squeezing in a healthy social and spiritual life for yourself. If you add planning meals, exercising, checking blood sugar, taking medication, and going to regular doctor appointments, you might feel like you're slipping into a state of no return.

There are a couple of strategies to help you. First, sit with your daily calendar to see how to fit all of it in. Maybe your family will need to pitch in more. If you're the one who takes the brunt of the chores, I encourage you to get strong and be clear that the extra time you need to take care of yourself is important to your health not only today but also tomorrow, next month, and in the future. If you're the primary chauffeur to the mall, movies, and piano practice, your kids may balk that you're not able to pick them up after all of their activities because you're now going to the gym regularly. Stick to your self-care routine. It won't take long for them to know that Mom is serious about her diabetes. They'll learn to adjust their schedules, too.

Speaking of the kids, why not ask them to cook dinner a couple of nights a week if they're old enough? It doesn't have to be fancy, but it should be high on veggies, medium on protein, and low on carbs. Learning to cook a quick dinner (and cleaning the kitchen afterward) is a good skill for any teenager to have.

Self-care takes time. If you've been the chief housekeeper and it now feels like an extra burden, ask for some help. As long as kids are old enough to hold a dust rag, they can probably help you clean the house. If they're big enough to skillfully kick a soccer ball, they're old enough to push a vacuum. Make cleaning the house a family project. Remember that old saying, "Many hands make light work." Again, if you're feeling stressed about all you have to do around the house, find a way to lighten the load. Relieve the stress because stress makes diabetes harder to control.

If you still feel overwhelmed with all there is to do, it's time to prioritize. Make a list of five absolute priorities, and then list five things you and the family are willing to drop from the to-do list. If you like to see a movie every weekend, maybe it's time to scale it back to every other weekend. If you have been going to the school every week to volunteer time with kids, could that be scaled back? Maybe instead of taking two night classes a semester to further your education, you only take one. Whatever your situation, if you are feeling overburdened, you must learn to say "No" to some of the many requests you're faced with. I promise that you will be amazed at the power that comes from simplifying your life.

MOOD SWINGS

If you experience mood swings, especially at first, understand that it's normal. Sometimes the crankiness may be due to low blood sugar. Or you're frustrated at having to watch what you eat and unexpectedly snap at your spouse. Maybe your sister is nagging you because she thinks you're not making healthful food choices or are regularly skipping exercise class. These comments usually come from a place of love, but boy, can they be irritating!

This is where you get to practice the art of communication. Talk it through. Be open. If your husband repeatedly comments about you not going to exercise class, by talking about how his comments bug you, you actually may discover you don't really like that aerobics class anyway. Perhaps a 30-minute after-dinner walk is more to your liking. If your wife is nagging you about your diet, being open to her comments may reveal opportunities for improvement in your eating plan. Maybe your daily 4:30 p.m. binge is not weakness. It could indicate a blood sugar low you need to address—other than by eating a bag of chips.

EATING OUT

No one enjoys a great meal from a restaurant more than me. That experience, like so many others in my new world with diabetes, required some adjustments. Here are some tricks I learned so I could still enjoy great food while keeping my blood sugar in check:

★ Order soup (broth- or tomato-based) or salad (dressing on the side) before your meal. You will tend to eat less during the rest of the meal.

★ Don't fill up on bread. In fact, if a server brings bread to the table and no one wants it, ask that it be taken away.

★ Ask questions. Good restaurants can tell you how food is prepared and can make accommodations for people with special diets.

★ Try a restaurant with specific menu items designed with lower fat and calorie options.

★ Choose restaurants that specialize in fresh foods, and don't be afraid to try new things.

★ Ask the server to split your meal in half, with the second half packed to take with you. That way you never see it on your plate and have a great meal for later.

★ Avoid fast food restaurants. The food is notoriously unhealthy and if you are going to treat yourself to a meal out, go out, sit down, and make the experience last more than five minutes.

★ Split a plate of food with your dinner partner. Portions are so large at most restaurants that you still get a filling meal and save money to boot.

★ Get one dessert for the table and have only a bite or two instead of ordering a whole dessert for yourself.

TRAVELING WELL

As a person with diabetes, travel can be a big headache if you don't plan well. Below are some tips that should prove helpful whether you are going for a quick weekend getaway or halfway around the world for a month.

Mind your medications

Give your doctor a call before you cross time zones. Your medication schedule adjustments for travel can vary depending on what meds you are taking. Some oral medications work best when taken in the morning, and morning is suddenly evening when traveling from San Diego to Morocco. When traveling to different time zones, one of the best ways to make sure you take your oral medications on time is to use a wristwatch with an alarm. Let's say you live in Charlotte but are traveling to San Francisco for a quick business trip. Also suppose you take your medicine at nine o'clock every day. To remind you to take your medicine at the time your body is used to (East Coast time), set your wristwatch alarm to go off at what would normally be nine o'clock in Charlotte (six o'clock in San Francisco). Typically, if you take your meds morning and evening, you can vary your schedule and adjust a couple of hours one way or the other to compensate for time zone changes. But check with your doctor about varying your medication schedule. And definitely check with your doctor regarding medication schedules for a trip outside the United States where the time zone difference may be six hours or more.

Ask before you fly

Check with the airlines to find out if there are restrictions on carrying medical equipment on board. Airline security is tight, tight, tight. If you use insulin and syringes, refer to the Transportation Security Administration guidelines (www.tsa.gov) about packing a copy of your prescription, medical supplies, and needles in your carry-on. It also can't hurt to double-check with your airline about its policy, too. In today's world of heightened security, you need to follow directions to the letter in order to ensure you don't have any trouble getting to your gate.

Pack your snacks

Most carriers do not serve meals on flights of less than four hours, so it pays to take your own snacks. My favorite snacks are nutrition bars: There are many flavors (including low carb versions), they pack well, don't need refrigeration, are long-lasting, and are easily available at most any airport. Another good bring-along is peanut butter. Pre-packed squeeze tubes are perfect for a traveler. Also, cut fresh vegetables into bite-sized pieces and tote them along in a ziplock bag. I think it's always a good idea to bring your own healthy snacks when you travel but because of stringent security, check the latest guidelines from Transportation Security Administration Web site and your carrier before you fly.

Check the menu

If you're on a flight with meal service, call the airline a few days before your flight and request a diabetic meal—most airlines can accommodate this request. If they don't offer a diabetic meal, ask what the special meal options are, and choose what best fits your diet. Also, keep in mind that when you travel on an airplane (or bus, or train), you typically don't need to eat as much, as sitting in those cramped seats does not promote calorie burn.

Take it with you

Always bring your blood glucose monitor when you travel. You're on vacation but your diabetes is not. You're still responsible for daily monitoring and managing your blood sugar. Sometimes it is hard to tell the difference between low blood sugar and jet lag; measuring your blood sugar level will remove all doubt. Make sure to test your blood sugar often so you can best manage through the change of routine that traveling inevitably brings on.

Does anyone speak my language?

If you are traveling to a foreign country and don't speak the language, have some catch phrases written down that might help if you run into trouble. Some of these might include "I have diabetes," "I need sugar immediately," and "I need a doctor." It is also a good idea to have all your medications written down and with you at all times just in case you become unconscious. You may also consider wearing a medical alert bracelet. Last but not least, check with the hotel where you are staying or do an Internet search for local hospitals or clinics before you leave, just in case.

Avoid the buffet

One of the most tempting parts of travel is eating out, and nothing looks as good as a fine hotel's breakfast buffet. However, buffets are an invitation to overeat and drive your blood sugar beyond a healthy range. If you see something you simply can't resist, remember that almost every buffet item is also available from the restaurant's menu. It may cost a little more if you order it from the menu, but you get a set portion, making it harder to overeat.

Going on a cruise? They are famous for their buffets. Stick to your eating schedule and plan ahead. Know what an acceptable portion size is and stick to it. Eat vegetables with every meal. Avoid rich, creamy sauces. Imagine yourself before your cruise seeing all that the buffet has to offer and visualize yourself sticking to your plan. Share your plan with your travel partner, and ask him or her to keep an eye on you.

Find time to exercise

Carving out time for a calorie-burning activity can be difficult, especially when traveling for business. However, just a short, 30-minute walk is beneficial for the mind and body. Here are a few simple tricks I've used.

★ Stay at a hotel with a gym.

★ If you are staying in an unfamiliar area and want to exercise outdoors, always ask the hotel staff if you are in a safe neighborhood and if they can suggest walking or jogging routes. Some hotels even have maps available for just this purpose.

★ If it is safe, walk to your destination.

★ Take comfortable, quick-drying exercise clothes. You can wash them in your bathroom sink with a little Woolite (or hotel shampoo in a pinch). Remove excess water from the clothes by rolling them in a towel, and then hang them to dry. Most quick-drying clothes will air dry in two to three hours.

★ Keep snacks with you at all times in case of hypoglycemia.

Remember, when you adopt new habits for life, it doesn't matter if you are on a cruise, in your own kitchen, or at a state dinner with the president. You eat and exercise to support your life with diabetes.

CHAPTER 9

IT'S UP TO YOU

Being positive has taken me further in life than being negative. Being positive, however, does not mean I stick my head in the sand. That's why I took some time to learn about how diabetes could affect me if I ignored it. Here are three of the most important things I learned.

Truth # 1: It takes time to take care of yourself

There are still times when I wish that I didn't have the responsibility of watching almost everything that goes in my mouth and exercising. Fortunately, those burdensome days occur less frequently now than when I was first diagnosed. But they still happen. When I feel overwhelmed, all I want to do is go back to my old habits.

When my emotions start leading me down that path, I consciously engage my brain and body to break the emotional cycle. I take a walk, get on my elliptical trainer, or do something else physical. If you find yourself wanting to give in to your cravings, please don't. Borrow the techniques presented in this book for getting physical, use other tips and tricks that you learned in your diabetes education class, or come up with a few of your own. The important thing is to listen to what your feelings are telling you while avoiding the old, harmful behaviors.

Yes, the daily routine of blood sugar monitoring, eating several small meals, and getting enough exercise can be a chore on certain days. But I challenge you to consider how much more of a chore it will be to take care of yourself when blindness or other serious illnesses creep in.

Truth # 2: Unchecked diabetes can harm many bodily systems

Unfettered high blood sugar hurts a lot of your body, including the heart and blood vessels. Too much glucose can harden the arteries, which can lead to heart attack and/or stroke. Constant high blood sugar also clogs the tiny vessels feeding areas such as the kidneys, eyes, and nerves. Inadequate circulation leads to kidney damage (nephropathy), eye damage (retinopathy), and nerve damage (neuropathy).

Truth # 3: You don't have to end up like Great Grandpa Angus

A couple of generations ago, nobody made the link that if people with diabetes kept blood sugar levels as close to normal as possible, then they could slow or possibly prevent the progression of kidney, eye, heart, and nerve problems. That connection was finally and firmly established with two landmark clinical studies. The Diabetes Control and Complication Trial (DCCT)[21] followed more than 1,400 people with type 1 diabetes for a decade. By strictly controlling their blood sugar levels, study participants reduced the chance of developing eye disease by more than 75 percent, kidney disease by about half, and nerve disease by 60 percent.

The United Kingdom Prospective Diabetes Study (UKPDS) enrolled more than 5,100 people with type 2 diabetes throughout England, Northern Ireland, and Scotland. The 20-year trial showed that improved control of blood sugar levels decreased major diabetic eye disease by 25 percent and early kidney damage by approximately one third. For many of the patients with high blood pressure, getting that down reduced the risk of strokes by more than one third.[22]

These studies showed without a doubt that people with diabetes who kept their blood sugar as close to normal levels as possible had significantly less nerve damage, kidney disease, and eye damage. Keeping blood pressure under control, too, reduced the chances of having a stroke.

So, yes, you have quite an advantage over your great grandparents. They didn't know they could do anything to prevent serious complications from diabetes. You do.

A WORD OF CAUTION

You can make significant strides in preventing complications from diabetes. But for reasons totally out of your control—age, race, and genetic makeup—you might end up with some complications sooner or later. If this happens, know that developing complications may bring up feelings similar to ones that you had when you were first diagnosed: anger, denial, guilt, fear, and perhaps an overwhelming sense of, "Why me? AGAIN!" These feelings are normal. The principles you're learning now—diet, exercise, medications, working with your healthcare team, and turning to your support network— will continue to serve you if complications later arise.

CARDIOVASCULAR DISEASE

Cardiovascular disease accounts for more than 65 percent of all death among people with diabetes. We're also two to four times more likely to have a stroke. Although those statistics are distressing, just because you have diabetes doesn't mean you will have a heart attack or stroke. It does mean, however, that taking care of yourself now will make a significant difference in your quality of life down the line.

Hardening and narrowing of the arteries

First, a couple of definitions for you. *Arterio*sclerosis is a fancy word that means that arteries are getting stiff and thick. *Athero*sclerosis specifically refers to the narrowing of arteries due to plaque. When plaque builds inside arteries, there is less room for blood to flow. Think of plaque as a pimple-like growth that is a deposit of cholesterol inside an artery wall. Over time, a blood clot could form in that area and may eventually lead to a heart attack. One of the reasons heart disease is so much more of a risk for people with diabetes is, again, due to high blood sugar. Extra glucose in the blood can make the fats in the blood super sticky, which means blood vessels are more apt to get clogged. Getting your blood sugar within range and eating limited amounts of fat can help prevent clogging and narrowing of your blood vessels.

High blood pressure

High blood pressure (hypertension) plays a big role in heart disease. In fact, more than half of those with type 2 diabetes experience high blood pressure. Because it doesn't have any symptoms, you might not know that you have high blood pressure until you are tested by your doctor.

High blood pressure means your heart is pumping harder than it must. This extra pressure can hurt the linings of arteries, eventually leading to a narrowing or blockage. Left untreated, high blood pressure can injure the smaller vessels leading to organs such as the kidneys and eyes, leading to kidney disease or glaucoma.

Steps to reduce the chances of developing heart disease

To help prevent long-term vessel disease, you can control blood sugar levels and stop smoking. If you have high cholesterol, lifestyle modifications such as more exercise and less intake of saturated fat may do the trick. If not, your physician may prescribe cholesterol-lowering drugs.

Work to bring down high blood pressure, too. Your doctor will have appropriate recommendations, such as cutting down on salt and increasing exercise. Here's also where a registered dietitian or CDE can help create food and lifestyle strategies for you to reduce blood pressure. If you're unable to bring down blood pressure through changing your exercise and eating routines, your doctor may prescribe medication.

HEART ALERT

Your body gives you warning signs of what could turn out to be a life-threatening heart problem. If you experience any of these, call 9-1-1 or see your doctor right away:

★ Chest pain/discomfort

★ Pain in arms, jaw, neck, back, or stomach

★ Shortness of breath

★ Sweating

★ Light-headedness

★ Nausea

★ Fatigue

Women, like men, can have heart attack symptoms of chest pain or discomfort. But it's more common for women to have other warning signs, especially shortness of breath, pain in the back or jaw, or nausea and/or vomiting.

KIDNEY DISEASE

You can markedly reduce your risk of kidney disease by reducing high blood sugar levels. Between 10–20 percent of those with diabetes have kidney disease. Nearly 45 percent of new cases of kidney failure are due to diabetes. Serious kidney disease is more common among those with type 1 diabetes than those with type 2 diabetes.

Your two kidneys clean your blood several times each day. In the simplest terms, kidneys filter the blood to get waste out while keeping the nutrients, such as protein, in. Over time, it's normal for the kidneys to work a little less efficiently. It simply happens to all of us due to age. But when blood sugar levels remain continually high, the rate of this normal change rapidly increases. Severe kidney damage can result, meaning that kidneys keep more of the harmful waste in while letting the good stuff out.

Steps to reduce chances of developing kidney disease

Although diabetes can hurt your kidneys, you can do a lot to prevent long-term kidney damage. The most important thing you can do is keep your blood sugar under control. The DCCT study, mentioned at the beginning of this chapter, clearly showed that those who kept their blood sugar under control greatly reduced their risk of developing kidney disease. Also, if you have high blood pressure, get it under control because high blood pressure can damage your hard-working kidneys.

KIDNEY ALERT

Kidneys are vital to your continued good health because they help clean out the body's waste, and they are at special risk because of diabetes. Get to a doctor quickly if you experience the following:

★ Fluid retention (excessive swelling, puffiness, or bloating)

★ Fatigue and loss of sleep

★ Loss of appetite

★ Indigestion

★ Weakness

★ Inability to concentrate

EYE DISEASE

The innermost part of your eyeball is the delicate, white retina. It contains millions of receptor cells that respond to light. Light passes through the outer structures of the eye to converge in the retina. The retina then transmits signals through the optic nerve into a particular area of the brain. If your retinas are damaged, then so is the quality of your pictures. Damage to the eye (retinopathy) is a result of injury to the tiny blood vessels that lead to the retina.

All people with diabetes—both type 1 and type 2—are at risk for retinopathy. Between 40–45 percent of Americans diagnosed with diabetes have some stage of diabetic retinopathy. After 20 years with diabetes, nearly everyone with type 1 diabetes exhibits signs of retinopathy and most with type 2 diabetes show some symptoms of retinopathy. Those with diabetes are four times more likely to end up blind compared to those without diabetes.

Steps to reduce chances of developing diabetic retinopathy

There is a lot you can do to keep this disease from hindering your eyesight. If retinopathy is detected early on, you have a good chance of slowing its development or stopping it in its tracks. Here are three important steps:

1. Get an annual eye examination. Your eye doctor should give your eyes a thorough going over, including examining your eyes through dilated pupils.

2. Keep your blood sugar levels as close to normal as possible. The DCCT trial clearly showed that lowering blood glucose reduces the likelihood of developing this complication.

3. Work with your doctor to get high blood pressure under control. High blood pressure can worsen already existing eye problems.

Glaucoma

Since you have diabetes, you also have a higher chance than people without diabetes of developing glaucoma. Risk of developing glaucoma increases the longer someone has diabetes, and also with age. Glaucoma is a result of pressure that builds up in the eye. This pressure eventually pinches the tiny vessels that transport blood to the retina and optic nerve. Both drugs and surgery can be used to treat glaucoma.

Cataracts

Many people get cataracts, but those of us with diabetes are about 60 percent more likely to develop this condition. Diabetes also means we have a chance of developing them at a younger age, and that they might progress faster compared to people without diabetes. A cataract is a condition in which light is blocked from entering the eye because the lens becomes cloudy. In cases of mild cataracts, people can wear sunglasses to help protect the eyes; and if they already wear glasses, they can use glare-control lenses. For more severe cases, lens surgery may be an option.

EYE ALERT

Having your eyes examined once a year by an eye care professional is essential. If you experience any of the following symptoms, *don't wait* until your next scheduled eye exam. Get in right away.

★ Blurry vision

★ Difficulty in reading

★ Eye pain

★ Ongoing redness

★ Pressure in the eyes

★ Spots or floaters

NERVE DISEASE AND DAMAGE

Your nervous system is the master controller and communicator of your entire body. The nervous system sends and receives billions of electrical and chemical signals, telling cells in your body what to do. Nervous system signals are fast, specific, and usually generate an almost immediate response. Just as with the heart, kidneys, and eyes, high blood sugar levels over time can wreak havoc on the nerves. Good glucose control over the years can go a long way in preventing nerve damage.

Diabetes can foul up these communication lines to the point where the peripheral nerves—the communication wires that connect your brain and spinal cord to the rest of you—may no longer be able to transmit signals, or the signals may be transmitted at the wrong time or sent too slowly.

Nerve damage due to diabetes is called diabetic neuropathy. It can show up in a variety of ways, including pain or loss of sensation in the feet or hands. Bladder or bowel control may be an issue. Sexual dysfunction can also result. There may be general muscle weakness or a loss of sensation. While these conditions may be the result of diabetic neuropathy, they could also be from other causes not related to high blood sugar levels. If you experience any of them, be sure to see your physician.

Diabetic neuropathy can be painful

It's not clear why high blood sugar levels over a sustained period of time damage the nerves. It could be that excessive amounts of glucose disturb the chemicals within the nerves. Perhaps glucose-coated proteins cause the harm, or the blood supplies to the nerves may be limited. Or it could be that glucose does not directly affect the nerves. Rather, other bodily systems may be impacted by high blood sugar that adversely impacts the nerves.

Getting blood sugar levels under control can help you relieve symptoms if you have neuropathy, or avoid it entirely if you don't. However, if control of your blood sugar level remains poor for a long period, you are more likely to end up with symptoms of diabetic neuropathy.

Steps to reduce the chances of developing neuropathy

If you have symptoms of early neuropathy, tight control of your blood sugar can go a long way in preventing further damage. Doctors tend to recommend three things when neuropathy rears its head: Reach and maintain your optimum, healthy weight; Exercise regularly; and Manage blood sugar levels.

NERVE ALERT

Your nerves will give you warning signs of possible damage due to diabetes. Contact your doctor if you experience the following:

★ Numbness or tingling, especially in the feet

★ Pain, particularly in the hands, feet, or legs

I TAKE IT SERIOUSLY

I take diabetes seriously because I've learned what it can do to me if it goes unchecked. I figure I've got at least 40 years to go, and I'm planning on making the most of the next four decades. My plans don't include battling eye disease, kidney problems, heart ailments, or painful nerves. Yes, I get a little weary of having to be vigilant about exercise and diet. There are occasional days when I simply don't want to take care of myself. Even when that mood strikes, I still eat the right foods, exercise, and measure my blood sugar. I've been at this long enough to know that the mood will pass in a day or two (at the most). I always come out the other side, knowing that I've built the knowledge and discipline to manage this illness even when I don't want to play the game anymore. I stay in the game because, truth be told, diabetes has been my blessing in disguise.

CHAPTER 10

IT'S YOUR TURN

I have had quite a journey, thanks to diabetes. I have learned so much, and yet there is still so much more to know. It seems that almost daily there is a new clinical study, a new drug therapy, or a promising treatment that could be a boon to all of us. My initial feeling of emptiness and loss after diagnosis has since evolved into a process of learning, adapting, and sharing.

Taking control can be a challenge, especially in this society of instant gratification. For a person with diabetes, there is the easy way (the hamburger drive-through is right around the corner and will take less than three minutes), and there is the right way (planning daily meals to significantly reduce your need for a drive-through). Diabetes management is not always easy, but it can be done right.

THE TOP 10

To help myself do it right, I came up with a list of 10 must dos. I refer to them as my Top 10 Commandments of living with type 2 diabetes.

1. Thou shalt check blood sugar regularly.

2. Thou shalt eat a healthy diet and understand the value of nutrition.

3. Thou shalt engage the assistance of a healthcare team.

4. Thou shalt create and follow a diabetes management plan.

5. Thou shalt not smoke.

6. Thou shalt recognize the symptoms of low blood sugar and act accordingly.

7. Thou shalt exercise regularly.

8. Thou shalt create a positive environment.

9. Thou shalt share information with family and friends.

10. Thou shalt ask for help when needed.

KEEPING MY SPIRITS UP

After I got over the shock of my diagnosis, I found myself psyched up for the first six months or so. I was ready to conquer my new world. I was going to fight this thing, and I was going to beat it! After the newness wore off, I had some tough days. There were days when I wanted to pretend my diabetes did not exist. In fact, I did pretend a few times. Yet, I could not eat all I wanted without guilt.

Days of discouragement still happen, though much less frequently. Sometimes I just need someone with a friendly ear to let me get it off my chest. Other times, if the feeling lasts for more than two days, I force myself to sit down and write out what is frustrating me and what action I can take. Getting things on paper can be a real eye-opener. Not too long ago, I was feeling down in the dumps about having diabetes, and I started writing out my feelings. Turns out that my real problem was stress from dealing with people at a mortgage office during that time. I was on edge, and I had mislabeled diabetes as the source of my temporary woes. Just writing down a few actions I could take to alleviate stress during this time helped me pull through.

One of the most important aspects of managing diabetes is that successful management is a series of small steps that you take every day. Those little things you do every day, like learning to write things down to get them off your chest so you don't end up eating half a bag of cookies to make yourself feel better, will add up to big changes over a lifetime. Managing diabetes is an evolution, not a revolution.

Here are some examples: When I don't feel like exercising, I force myself to go out and walk (or go to the gym, or get on my bike) and commit to just 10 minutes of activity. Even on my worst days, I can exercise for 10 minutes. Then, after 10 minutes, I assess whether I want to go for a while longer or stop. I have used this trick dozens of times over the past several years, and only once did I stop after just 10 minutes. An object in motion tends to stay in motion; once your body and brain get warmed up, they like to keep going.

I have also learned little mental tricks while I am exercising to keep pushing myself those last few minutes. For instance, sometimes I imagine I am in a race, and I can hear the crowd cheering me on. Or, I think of my body as a mine of energy and when I am working out hard, I imagine that miners are digging away at my fat cells and feeding them to the "fire in my belly." Just like a locomotive running on coal, the fire gets hotter, and I go faster with every shovelful of fat I feed to the fire. I imagine running fast and the fat falling away from my body, making my physical efforts seem as easy as kindergarten math.

Here is another great trick. When you lose a little weight, find something equivalent to the weight you lost and carry it around for five minutes. When you lose five pounds, carry around a bag of sugar and think of how great it is not to have to carry that around your belly or thighs anymore. After I lost 20 pounds, I carried a 20-pound barbell around the gym for a few minutes. It was both exhilarating and exhausting—exhilarating because I could really feel in my hands how much weight was gone, and exhausting because lugging around 20 extra pounds is not easy.

MORE THAN DIET AND EXERCISE

Because diabetes is a lifelong condition, it's important to look at it as more than diet, exercise, and medication. Look at your whole self—mind, body, and spirit—and make sure those elements are in balance. If you are following traditional Western medicine, your doctor will typically focus on the body and the numbers that help a physician to track your progress (your blood sugar levels, weight, HbA1c, etc.).

I believe you need to focus on the other things that make you feel your best. You must be your own best advocate and treat yourself as number one. If your child were ill, you would give him all your energy to ensure a strong recovery. Why not pour that same passion and energy into your diabetes management? After all, you are worth the effort! Here are some suggestions that should bolster your body, mind, and spirit.

Massage

Almost nothing feels better than a professional massage. Massage aids in circulation, relaxes your mind and body, and works out muscle aches. If you don't regularly get massages, ask for referrals from friends or family. If you are trying a massage for the first time, or you are switching to a new massage therapist, ask for someone who has at least three years of experience.

If you need to keep expenses in check, see if there is an accredited school of massage in your area. Most massage schools offer a variety of services for about half the usual cost. (You can look up massage therapy schools in your area by visiting www.naturalhealers.com.)

Aromatherapy

Aromatherapy does not cure disease. However, your sense of smell is strong, and as you deeply inhale different scents, your body may have a very positive reaction. Here are some examples provided by the National Association of Holistic Aromatherapy:[23]

★ Lavender aids in relaxation.

★ Peppermint helps relieve indigestion and muscle aches.

★ Eucalyptus helps enhance the immune system and assists in alleviating muscle tension.

★ Roman chamomile promotes relaxation and may relieve sleeplessness and anxiety.

★ Rosemary helps stimulate mental processes, as well as the immune system.

I use aromatherapy in a number of ways. I pack a small bottle of lavender essential oil in my purse when traveling. If you have been on a plane recently, you know that the recycled air combined with all those closely packed people can be nasty for the nostrils. I put a drop of lavender oil under my nose, close my eyes, and breathe deeply. It really does take my mind off the stress of travel for a while.

I also use aromatherapy at the end of a meal, to help my brain refocus from the smell of food to other things. Both the scent of geranium and citrus are uplifting yet relaxing.

To learn more about aromatherapy, start with the National Association for Holistic Aromatherapy (NAHA, www.naha.org). Also, check with your local library or bookseller, as there are many great books on this subject.

Yoga

Yoga has held two notable benefits for me. First, yoga has helped me physically. The postures work my muscles, improve my flexibility, and I believe yoga has boosted my immune system. Secondly, when doing yoga, I have to concentrate so hard on the poses that all other thoughts, worries, and distractions leave my mind, if only for that hour. It is the only activity I have found so far that allows me to completely forget for one hour that I have diabetes. For me, that is really saying something.

STARTING YOUR JOURNEY

Since being diagnosed, I have lost 40 pounds—and kept it off. This is the first time I've not yo-yoed back to a heavier, unhealthy weight. I have taken the initiative to manage my disease and to create a healthcare team around me. Just as importantly, I've learned how and when to ask for help.

Most amazingly, though, diabetes has given me focus. It has taught me about discipline and given me the perspective to concentrate on what I really want to accomplish. I plan to spend the rest of my life, both personally and professionally, working with people with diabetes who might need a helping hand and a caring attitude.

Earlier, I mentioned I wanted to beat my diabetes. But I've learned that all that fighting leads to nothing but exhaustion. So, I've changed my outlook. Rather than looking at diabetes as something to beat, I choose to incorporate it into my life and accept the fact that I have a chronic illness. I've learned to take control without all that mental and emotional battle. You, too, can take control. You can live healthfully and have a long, productive life with diabetes. By making small changes every day, it will add up to big results over the long haul.

In the end, it all boils down to *action*. What action will you take today to better control your diabetes? After all, it is action that drives inspiration. And that is what I want for you, to live an inspired life. Through action, you can control your diabetes and create a positive environment for yourself and others. You can inspire your family, your friends, and your healthcare team. So take action, inspire those you care about most, and live your life to the fullest. The world is knocking on your door. Are you ready to answer?

50 LITTLE THINGS YOU CAN DO TO BETTER MANAGE YOUR DIABETES

I am all for using tips and tricks to make my life easier. And that includes managing my diabetes. Below are 50 actions that work for me, sorted into three categories so you can quickly skim the list and start applying them today. Once you've made three or four a part of your regular routine, add three or four more. Keep going. Before you know it, you'll be a master manager of your diabetes and your life.

EXERCISE

1. Work out with a buddy.

2. Put a towel over the clock of your cardio machine—it makes the time pass faster.

3. Use a heart rate monitor.

4. Schedule workout appointments for yourself. If your calendar says you work out at 6 p.m., then keep that appointment with yourself.

5. Invest in a new pair of tennis shoes.

6. Get a subscription to a health or exercise magazine.

7. Work out in light, comfortable clothes.

8. Pick a qualified personal trainer for weight training, and be sure he or she is certified by any of the top three fitness organizations: the National Strength and Conditioning Association, the American Council on Exercise, or the American College of Sports Medicine.

9. Try a new activity at least three times before you decide you hate it.

10. Know your current physical state. If you have not exercised in some time, train for a while before you attempt to hike up the Grand Canyon.

11. Go for a walk with your kids. If you don't have kids, get a dog and walk with it or borrow a friend's dog for regular power walks.

12. Enter yourself in a charity walk/run.

13. If you sleep eight hours a night, there are 32 half hours remaining in the rest of the day. Can you spare one of those half hours for fitness? Make a personal exercise plan, and schedule your half hour right now.

DIET

14. Eat a salad before dinner every night. It fills you up, and you get your greens at the same time.

15. Think before you drink. There are 4 grams of sugar in a teaspoon. When you want to drink a soda that contains 40 grams of sugar, that means you're consuming 10 teaspoons of sugar. Ridiculous!

16. Drink diet soda rather than regular.

17. Better yet, drink green tea. It contains antioxidants that help your body ward off illnesses.

18. When eating out, tell the waitperson to box up half your meal before bringing it to the table. That way, you only eat half the meal. Save the other half for a different meal.

19. Beware of condiments like mayonnaise or sour cream—they are usually packed with calories and fat. Salsa and mustard are your best choices.

20. Drink at least eight glasses of water every day.

21. Keep a food log and count your calories. Depending on size and activity level, women should typically stay between 1,500–2,000 calories, and men between 2,000–2,500. Work with your doctor or nutritionist to learn *your* ideal intake.

22. Reduce the amount of red meat in your diet. If you have a choice, pick lean chicken or turkey instead.

23. Beware of cold cereal. Try to find a brand where sugar is not one of the first three ingredients. Plain old sugar is disguised under many names: high fructose corn syrup, fructose, or sucrose.

24. Don't overdo alcohol. A 4-ounce glass of wine contains about 80 calories.

25. All alone and want to eat when you are not hungry? Call a long-lost friend instead and spend an hour getting caught up.

26. Eat more fresh fish.

27. Subscribe to a healthy cooking magazine.

28. Become a vegetarian for a week.

29. Take a cooking class that focuses on meals that are friendly to those with diabetes.

30. Put a list on your fridge of 10 approved snacks. That way, if you get hungry, you can look at a list and immediately make a better choice, rather than reaching for the first thing you see.

31. Set up a contest with your friends or family to see who can make the best diabetic-friendly dish. Then have a potluck dinner.

DAILY LIFE

32. Stand up straight—it will make you look stronger and leaner.

33. Practice balance, moderation, and variation.

34. Create your positive environment and share it with others.

35. Smile at others when walking down the street. See how many people smile back.

36. Volunteer.

37. Reduce your stress levels. Start by thinking positive thoughts.

38. Indulge in a spa treatment.

39. Develop a plan for your diabetes management, and set challenging yet reasonable goals.

40. Celebrate your accomplishments.

41. Turn off your TV for an hour and be physically active instead.

42. Use what motivates you. (I have a friend who is trying to lose weight. She carries around a picture of herself from 1999 when she was 40 pounds lighter. She looks at it before every meal.)

43. Get enough sleep.

44. Avoid comparing yourself to others. You are unique and must do what works for you.

45. Try something new.

46. Identify your moods, both good and bad. Learn your triggers and how to deal with them.

47. Spend time with friends and family.

48. Increase your laughing by 100 percent.

49. Graciously accept compliments.

50. Learn to be at peace with yourself.

APPENDIX 2

CHARTS TO MEASURE YOUR PROGRESS

★ Daily Fasting Blood Sugar

★ Daily Food, Blood Sugar, and Activity Log

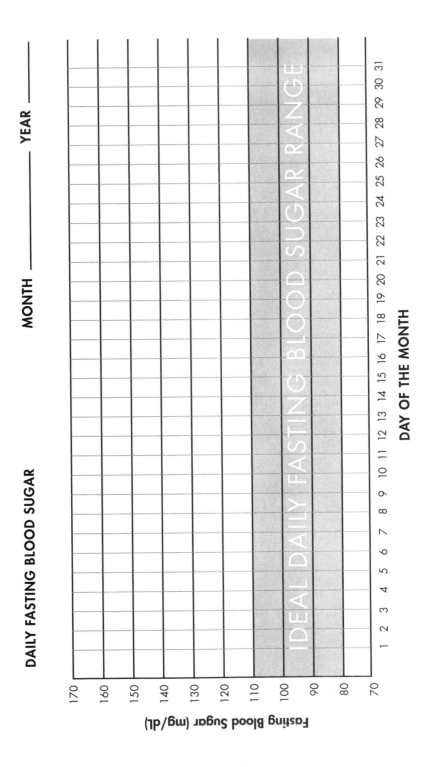

DAILY FASTING BLOOD SUGAR

MONTH ——————— YEAR ———————

Fasting Blood Sugar (mg/dL)

170 160 150 140 130 120 110 100 90 80 70

IDEAL DAILY FASTING BLOOD SUGAR RANGE

DAY OF THE MONTH

1 2 3 4 5 6 7 8 9 10 11 12 13 14 15 16 17 18 19 20 21 22 23 24 25 26 27 28 29 30 31

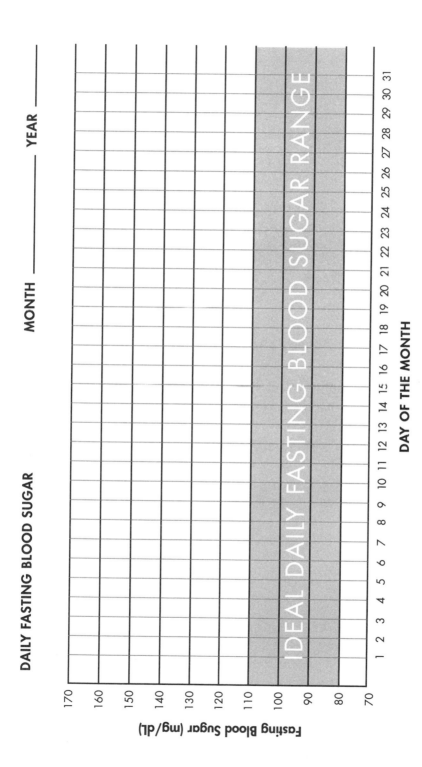

DAILY FASTING BLOOD SUGAR

MONTH ——— YEAR ———

Fasting Blood Sugar (mg/dL)

170 160 150 140 130 120 110 100 90 80 70

IDEAL DAILY FASTING BLOOD SUGAR RANGE

DAY OF THE MONTH

1 2 3 4 5 6 7 8 9 10 11 12 13 14 15 16 17 18 19 20 21 22 23 24 25 26 27 28 29 30 31

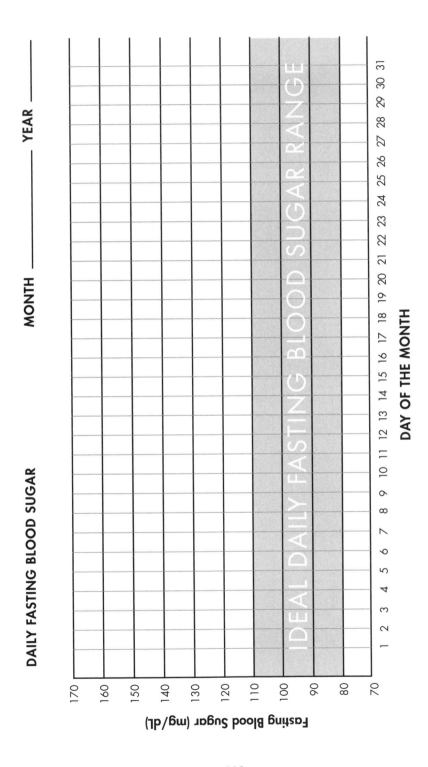

DATE _____

DAILY FOOD, BLOOD SUGAR, AND ACTIVITY LOG

TIME	FOOD	CARBS	BLOOD SUGAR (mg/dL)	EXERCISE
6:00 a.m.				
6:30 a.m.				
7:00 a.m.				
7:30 a.m.				
8:00 a.m.				
8:30 a.m.				
9:00 a.m.				
9:30 a.m.				
10:00 a.m.				
10:30 a.m.				
11:00 a.m.				
11:30 a.m.				
12:00 p.m.				
12:30 p.m.				
1:00 p.m.				
1:30 p.m.				
2:00 p.m.				
2:30 p.m.				
3:00 p.m.				

TIME	FOOD	CARBS	BLOOD SUGAR (mg/dL)	EXERCISE
3:30 p.m.				
4:00 p.m.				
4:30 p.m.				
5:00 p.m.				
5:30 p.m.				
6:00 p.m.				
6:30 p.m.				
7:00 p.m.				
7:30 p.m.				
8:00 p.m.				
8:30 p.m.				
9:00 p.m.				
9:30 p.m.				
10:00 p.m.				
10:30 p.m.				
11:00 p.m.				
Total				

Notes:

DATE _____

DAILY FOOD, BLOOD SUGAR, AND ACTIVITY LOG

TIME	FOOD	CARBS	BLOOD SUGAR (mg/dL)	EXERCISE
6:00 a.m.				
6:30 a.m.				
7:00 a.m.				
7:30 a.m.				
8:00 a.m.				
8:30 a.m.				
9:00 a.m.				
9:30 a.m.				
10:00 a.m.				
10:30 a.m.				
11:00 a.m.				
11:30 a.m.				
12:00 p.m.				
12:30 p.m.				
1:00 p.m.				
1:30 p.m.				
2:00 p.m.				
2:30 p.m.				
3:00 p.m.				

TIME	FOOD	CARBS	BLOOD SUGAR (mg/dL)	EXERCISE
3:30 p.m.				
4:00 p.m.				
4:30 p.m.				
5:00 p.m.				
5:30 p.m.				
6:00 p.m.				
6:30 p.m.				
7:00 p.m.				
7:30 p.m.				
8:00 p.m.				
8:30 p.m.				
9:00 p.m.				
9:30 p.m.				
10:00 p.m.				
10:30 p.m.				
11:00 p.m.				
Total				

Notes:

DATE _____

DAILY FOOD, BLOOD SUGAR, AND ACTIVITY LOG

TIME	FOOD	CARBS	BLOOD SUGAR (mg/dL)	EXERCISE
6:00 a.m.				
6:30 a.m.				
7:00 a.m.				
7:30 a.m.				
8:00 a.m.				
8:30 a.m.				
9:00 a.m.				
9:30 a.m.				
10:00 a.m.				
10:30 a.m.				
11:00 a.m.				
11:30 a.m.				
12:00 p.m.				
12:30 p.m.				
1:00 p.m.				
1:30 p.m.				
2:00 p.m.				
2:30 p.m.				
3:00 p.m.				

TIME	FOOD	CARBS	BLOOD SUGAR (mg/dL)	EXERCISE
3:30 p.m.				
4:00 p.m.				
4:30 p.m.				
5:00 p.m.				
5:30 p.m.				
6:00 p.m.				
6:30 p.m.				
7:00 p.m.				
7:30 p.m.				
8:00 p.m.				
8:30 p.m.				
9:00 p.m.				
9:30 p.m.				
10:00 p.m.				
10:30 p.m.				
11:00 p.m.				
Total				

Notes:

APPENDIX 3

RESOURCES

AMERICAN DIABETES ASSOCIATION
www.diabetes.org
800-DIABETES (800-342-2383)

JOSLIN DIABETES CENTER
www.joslin.org
617-732-2400

NATIONAL DIABETES INFORMATION CLEARINGHOUSE (NDIC)
diabetes.niddk.nih.gov
800-860-8747

INTERNATIONAL DIABETES FEDERATION
www.idf.org
Brussels, Belgium
+32-2-53855111

AMERICAN ASSOCIATION OF DIABETES EDUCATORS (AADE)
www.diabeteseducator.org
800-338-3633

THE PHARMACEUTICAL RESEARCH AND MANUFACTURERS OF AMERICA (PHRMA)

www.phrma.org
202-835-3400

AMERICAN COUNCIL ON EXERCISE

www.acefitness.org
858-279-8227

DIABETES EXERCISE AND SPORTS ASSOCIATION

www.diabetes-exercise.org
800-898-4322

CENTERS FOR MEDICARE AND MEDICAID INFORMATION

www.cms.hhs.gov
800-MEDICARE (800-633-4227)

DAILY STRENGTH

dailystrength.org/support/Endocrine_System/Diabetes_Type_2

DEFEAT DIABETES FOUNDATION, INC.

www.defeatdiabetes.org

D LIFE

www.dlife.com

E-MAIL ALERTS

You can have the latest diabetes news sent directly to you every day via e-mail. Just go to www.google.com, and click "news alerts." Enter "type 2 diabetes" as the topic you wish to monitor, and then enter your e-mail address. Next thing you know, Google automatically searches for related articles and information on your behalf every day, and then e-mails the hyperlinks directly to you.

APPENDIX 4

GLOSSARY

Much of the information in this glossary is derived from the encyclopedia and dictionary found through Medline Plus (www.medlineplus.gov) and information from the National Diabetes Information Clearinghouse (www.diabetes.niddk.nih.gov).

A

Adrenaline (also called Epinephrine) – This is a catecholamine. Catecholamines are hormones produced by the adrenal glands, located at the top of the kidneys. They are released into the blood during times of physical or emotional stress.

Arteriosclerosis – A condition in which the walls of the arteries grow thick and hard.

Atherosclerosis – A form of arteriosclerosis in which fatty material collects along the inner walls of the arteries. This fatty material thickens, hardens, and may eventually block the arteries.

B

Blood Glucose Monitoring – A measurement of glucose (sugar) in the blood. The test can be done at any time on a portable machine. It can be a self-test for a person with diabetes.

BMI (Body Mass Index) – An estimate of how much you should weigh, based on your height. Here are the steps to calculate it:

★ Multiply your weight in pounds by 703.

★ Divide that answer by your height in inches.

★ Divide that answer by your height in inches, again.

For example, a woman who weighs 200 pounds and is 68 inches tall (5 feet, 8 inches) has a BMI of 30.4.

C

Carbohydrates – One of the main dietary components. The primary function of carbohydrates is to provide energy for the body, especially the brain and the nervous system.

Cataract – A cloudy or opaque area (an area you cannot see through) in the lens of the eye.

Complex Carbohydrates – These are made up of sugar molecules that are strung together in long, complex chains. Complex carbohydrates are found in foods such as peas, beans, whole grains, and vegetables. Both simple and complex carbohydrates are turned to glucose (blood sugar) in the body and are used as energy.

E

Endocrinology – A science dealing with the endocrine glands.

Endocrine Glands – Glands that release hormones into the bloodstream.

Epinephrine – See adrenaline.

Erectile Dysfunction – An erection problem is the inability to get or maintain an erection that is firm enough for a man to have intercourse. A man may be unable to get an erection at all, or may lose the erection during intercourse before he is ready. When this condition persists, the medical term is erectile dysfunction.

F

Fasting Blood Glucose Level – The amount of glucose measured in the blood after several hours of not eating, usually six to eight. Diabetes is diagnosed if the fasting blood glucose level is higher than 126 mg/dL on two occasions. Levels between 100–126 mg/dL are referred to as impaired fasting glucose or prediabetes.

G

Gene – A short piece of DNA, which tells the body how to build a specific protein. There are approximately 30,000 genes in each cell of the human body. The combination of all genes makes up the blueprint for the human body and its functions.

Gestational Diabetes – This is when high blood glucose develops at any time during pregnancy in a woman who does not otherwise have diabetes.

Glaucoma – This is a group of disorders that damage the optic nerve, which is the nerve that carries visual information from the eye to the brain. Damage to the optic nerve causes vision loss, which may progress to blindness. Most people with glaucoma have increased fluid pressure in the eye, a condition known as increased intraocular pressure.

Glucagon – A hormone that is produced by cells in the pancreas. It helps to regulate blood sugar levels. As the level of blood sugar is decreased, the pancreas releases more glucagon, and vice versa. The hormone stimulates the liver to release glucose.

Glucose – A major source of energy for most cells of the body, including those in the brain.

Growth Hormone – A hormone released by the pituitary gland, a small endocrine gland at the bottom of the brain near the base of the scull. Excess growth hormone can increase blood pressure and blood sugar.

H

HbA1c – A measure of average blood glucose during the previous 2–3 months. It is a very helpful way to determine how well diabetes treatment is working.

Hemoglobin – A protein in red blood cells that carries oxygen.

Hormone – A product of living cells that circulates in body fluids and produces a specific effect on the activity of cells some distance away.

Hyperglycemia – An excess of glucose in the blood.

Hypertension – Abnormally high blood pressure.

Hypoglycemia – Too little glucose in the blood. Hypoglycemia results when your body's glucose is used up too rapidly, when glucose is released into the bloodstream too slowly, or when too much insulin is released into the bloodstream.

I

Immune System – The system that protects the body from foreign substances, cells, and tissues by producing the immune response.

Impaired Fasting Glucose (IFG) – A condition in which the fasting blood sugar level is 100–125 milligrams per deciliter (mg/dL) after an overnight fast. The level is higher than normal but not high enough to be classified as diabetes. Also called prediabetes.

Impaired Glucose Tolerance (IGT) – A condition in which the blood sugar level is 140–199 mg/dL after a 2-hour oral glucose tolerance test. This level is higher than normal but not high enough to be classified as diabetes. Also called prediabetes.

Insulin – The role of insulin is to move glucose from the bloodstream into muscle, fat, and liver cells, where it can be used as fuel. It is produced by the pancreas in response to increased glucose levels in the blood.

Insulin Resistance – A condition in which your muscle, fat, and liver cells do not use insulin properly. The pancreas tries to keep up with the demand for insulin by producing more. Eventually, the pancreas cannot keep up with the body's need for insulin, and excess glucose builds up in the bloodstream.

Insulin-dependent Diabetes Mellitus – A former name for type 1 diabetes. This form of diabetes also used to be called juvenile diabetes.

J

Juvenile Diabetes – A former name for type 1 diabetes.

K

Ketoacidosis – This is a complication of diabetes. It is caused by the buildup of by-products of fat breakdown, called ketones. This occurs when glucose is not available as a fuel source for the body, and fat is used instead.

Ketone – Ketones are produced by the breakdown of fat and muscle, and they are harmful at high levels.

L

Lancet – A sharp-pointed and commonly two-edged instrument used to make small incisions, also called a lance.

Logbook – A written record of daily blood sugar readings and medications.

M

mg/dL – Milligrams per deciliter.

N

Nephropathy – Kidney disease. Diabetic kidney disease takes many years to develop. Overall, kidney damage rarely occurs in the first 10 years of diabetes, and usually 15–25 years will pass before kidney failure occurs. For people who live with diabetes for more than 25 years without any signs of kidney failure, the risk of ever developing it decreases.

Neuropathy – Diabetic neuropathies are a family of nerve disorders caused by diabetes. Neuropathies lead to numbness and sometimes pain and weakness in the hands, arms, feet, and legs. Problems may also occur in every organ system, including the digestive tract, heart, and sex organs.

O

Obesity – A condition that is characterized by excessive accumulation and storage of fat in the body and that in an adult is typically indicated by a body mass index of 30 or greater.

Oral Glucose Tolerance Test – This is the most common glucose tolerance test. Those taking the test cannot eat or drink anything for several hours before the test. Blood sugar is measured before drinking a liquid containing a certain amount of glucose. Blood sugar levels are then measured every 30–60 minutes after drinking the solution. The test takes up to 3 hours.

P

Pancreas – A large gland that lies behind the stomach. It secretes digestive enzymes that pass to the intestine to help breakdown proteins, fats, and carbohydrates. It also secretes the hormones insulin and glucagon.

Placenta – The temporary organ that develops during pregnancy and supports the fetus as it grows in the uterus.

Plaque – Fat, cholesterol, and other matter that build up in the walls of arteries to form hard substances.

Plasma – The pale yellow fluid portion of whole blood that consists of water and dissolved proteins, electrolytes, sugars, lipids, metabolic waste products, amino acids, hormones, and vitamins.

Postprandial – After a meal.

Prandial – Of or relating to a meal.

Prediabetes – People with blood glucose levels that are higher than normal but not yet in the diabetic range have prediabetes. Doctors sometimes call this condition impaired fasting glucose (IFG) or impaired glucose tolerance (IGT), depending on the test used to diagnose it.

Preprandial – Before a meal.

Q-T

Retinopathy – The retina is the lining at the back of the eye. The retina's job is to sense light coming into the eye. Retinas have tiny blood vessels that are easy to damage. Having high blood glucose and high blood pressure for a long time can damage these tiny blood vessels. Retinopathy is the medical term for this diabetes eye problem.

Risk Factor – Something that increases risk or susceptibility.

Type 1 Diabetes – A condition in which the body makes little or no insulin, and daily injections of insulin are needed to sustain life. This is usually diagnosed in childhood.

Type 2 Diabetes – This type of diabetes is far more common than type 1 and makes up most cases of diabetes. It usually occurs in adulthood. The pancreas does not make enough insulin to keep blood glucose levels normal, often because the body does not respond well to the insulin.

U–Z

Whole Blood – Blood with all its components, such as plasma, red blood cells, white blood cells (which fight disease), and platelets (which play a part in clotting).

ENDNOTES

[1] Centers for Disease Control and Prevention, Diabetes Public Health Resource, Data & Trends, Diabetes Surveillance System. http://www.cdc.gov/diabetes/statistics/age/fig1.htm.

[2] Reaney, P. Overweight urged to slim down to cut diabetes risk. *Reuters Health Information*. November 9, 2004.

[3] Diabetes 4-1-1: Facts, Figures, and Statistics at a Glance, American Diabetes Association, Inc. 2005.

[4] National Diabetes Information Clearinghouse (NDIC), Diagnosis of Diabetes. http://diabetes.niddk.nih.gov/dm/pubs/diagnosis/index.htm.

[5] Knowler WE, Barrett-Conner E, Fowler SE, et al., Reduction in the incidence of type 2 diabetes with lifestyle intervention or metformin. *N Engl J Med.* 2002 Feb 7; 346(6):393-403.

[6] American Diabetes Association, Standards of Medical Care in Diabetes—2007. *Diabetes Care.* Jan 2007; 30:S4-S41.

[7] American College of Endocrinology Consensus Statement on Guidelines for Glycemic Control. *Endocr Pract.* Jan/Feb 2002; 8(Suppl 1):5-11.

[8] U.S. Food and Drug Administration, "FDA Approves First Ever Inhaled Insulin Combination Product for Treatment of Diabetes." Jan 27, 2006. http://www.fda.gov/bbs/topics/news/2006/NEW01304.html.

[9] Your Healthcare Team, http://www.diabetes.org/whos-who-on-your-health-care-team/your-health-care-team.jsp. Copyright © 2006 American Diabetes Association from http://www.diabetes.org. Reprinted with permission from *The American Diabetes Association.*

[10] The American Psychological Association, "Coping with Serious Illness," http://www.apahelpcenter.org/articles/article.php?id=4. Reprinted with permission.

[11] Landolt MA, Ribi K, Laimbacher J, et al., Posttraumatic stress disorder in parents of children with newly diagnosed type 1 diabetes. *J Pediatr Pschol.* 2002 Oct-Nov; 27(7):647-52.

[12] Hegel MT, Moore CP, Collins ED, et al., Distress, psychiatric syndromes, and impairment of function in women with newly diagnosed breast cancer. *Cancer.* 2006 Dec 15; 107(12):2924-31.

[13] Landolt MA, Vollrath M, Laimbacher J, et al., Prospective study of posttraumatic stress disorder in parents of children with newly diagnosed type 1 diabetes. *J Am Acad Child Adolesc Psychiatry.* 2005 Jul; 44(7):682-9.

[14] Cotton Richard T., Lifestyle & Weight Management: Consultant Manual. San Diego: American Council on Exercise; 1996.

[15] Georgia State University Department of Kinesiology and Health, "The exercise and physical fitness page." http://www2.gsu.edu/~wwwfit/bodycomp.html.

[16] Adapted from Partnership for Healthy Weight Management, Consumer.gov. http://www.consumer.gov/weightloss/bmi.htm.

[17] Freeman J, "The glycemic index debate: does the type of carbohydrate really matter," http://www.diabetes.org/glycemic-index.jsp.

[18] Foster-Powell K, Holt SHA, Brand-Miller JC. International table of glycemic index and glycemic load values. *Am J Clin Nutr.* 2002;76:5–56. Reprinted with permission of J. Brand-Miller.

[19] American Dietetic Association, Visualize the Right Portion Size. http://www.eatright.org/cps/rde/xchg/ada/hs.xsl/home_4367_ENU_HTML.htm. Reprinted with permission from www.eatright.org.

[20] "You must unlearn what you have learned....Try not. Do. Or do not. There is no try." – Yoda. ©Lucasfilm Ltd. & TM. All rights reserved. Used under authorization.

[21] The Diabetes Control and Complications Trial Research Group. The Effect of Intensive Treatment of Diabetes on the Development and Progression of Long-Term Complications in Insulin-Dependent Diabetes Mellitus. *N Engl J Mcd.* September 1993; 329:977-986.

[22] University of Oxford, The Oxford Centre for Diabetes, Endocrinology & Metabolism, Diabetes Trial Unit, UK Prospective Diabetes Study. http://www.dtu.ox.ac.uk/index.php?maindoc=/ukpds/results.php.

[23] National Association for Holistic Aromatherapy, Top 10 Essential Oils. http://www.naha.org/top_10.htm. The National Association for Holistic Aromatherapy (NAHA), 3327 W. Indian Trail Road, PMB 144, Spokane, WA 99208 U.S.A. Reprinted with permission.

INDEX